BLACK BELT
HEALING

BLACK BELT HEALING

A Martial Artist's Guide to Pain Management and Injury Recovery

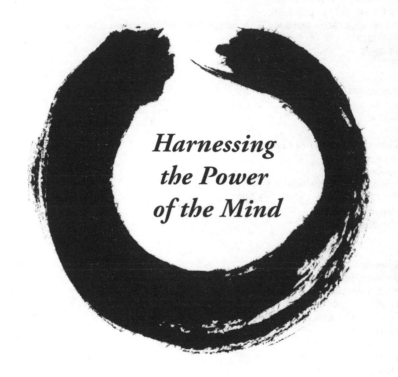

Harnessing the Power of the Mind

David Nelson, Ph.D.
Foreword by Stacey Shook, Ph.D.

TUTTLE PUBLISHING
Tokyo • Rutland, Vermont • Singapore

Published by Tuttle Publishing, an imprint of Periplus Editions (HK) Ltd., with editorial offices at 364 Innovation Drive, North Clarendon, Vermont 05759 U.S.A. and 61 Tai Seng Avenue, #02-12, Singapore 534167

Library of Congress Cataloging-in-Publication Data
Nelson, David, 1955-
 Black belt healing : harnessing the power of the mind / by David Nelson ; with a foreword by Stacey Shook.
   p. cm.
 Includes bibliographical references.
 ISBN 978-0-8048-4124-5 (pbk.)
 1. Mental healing. 2. Mind and body. 3. Martial arts--Psychological aspects. I. Title.
 RZ400.N44 2010
 615.8'515--dc22

                              2009028084

ISBN 978-0-8048-4124-5

Distributed by

North America, Latin America & Europe
Tuttle Publishing
364 Innovation Drive
North Clarendon, VT 05759-9436 U.S.A.
Tel: 1 (802) 773-8930; Fax: 1 (802) 773-6993
info@tuttlepublishing.com
www.tuttlepublishing.com

Japan
Tuttle Publishing
Yaekari Building, 3rd Floor
5-4-12 Osaki; Shinagawa-ku
Tokyo 141 0032
Tel: (81) 3 5437-0171; Fax: (81) 3 5437-0755
tuttle-sales@gol.com

Asia Pacific
Berkeley Books Pte. Ltd.
61 Tai Seng Avenue #02-12
Singapore 534167
Tel: (65) 6280-1330; Fax: (65) 6280-6290
inquiries@periplus.com.sg
www.periplus.com

14 13 12 11 10   6 5 4 3 2 1

Printed in Singapore

Contents

Acknowledgements

I wish to express my sincere appreciation to my wife, Jean, for her patience while I lived with a computer on my lap. I would also like to acknowledge and express appreciation to my daughter, Hannah, for the wonderful illustrations contained in this book. Also to:

Bob and Paula Nelson for their early editing of the book.
Master Stacey Shook for writing the foreword.
Jen and Dan Lutsey for their encouraging words.
Sandra Korinchak and Bud Sperry of Tuttle Publishing for their wonderful editing.
Shihan Paul Dean and Reverend Nonin Chowaney for their teachings and unending patience.

Note to the Reader
This book is not a substitute for appropriate medical care, but rather an adjunct to the medical treatment of pain. You should always consult a medical professional for the treatment of any injury or persistent pain.

Foreword

One of the definitions of journey is travel or passage from one place to another—also referred to as a trip. If we give the above definition some thought, we have already embarked on a journey of fourteen words. I love journeys. Our bodies may at times remain static, but our mind has "left the building." Even the most mundane of trips has imbedded within it the possibility of adventure. We miss many adventures because we fail to look through the "possibilities window." We then can experience the old saying, "I was at the train station when my ship came in." Learning to notice and realize that there are no ordinary moments sets the stage for learning new things.

Black Belt Healing is one of those special journeys that, given your attention, will bring the adventure into view. The "possibilities window" is accessible and we are able to start and see how and learn why the Art of Mind-Swords works towards healing: first with necessary guidance and later quite independently. Dr. David Nelson has successfully brought to life the Art of Mind-Swords through his knowledge, creativity, use of language, and visualization! The techniques and strategies are presented in an easy to follow, systematic process that allows the practitioner to utilize the material contained in this book.

As a long-time martial artist and Ph.D. psychotherapist, I have worked to bring psychology and martial arts together. This has not always been an easy task due to the differences in Eastern and Western philosophies of energy flow and power of thought. The dojo or training place is an ideal platform for the meeting of these somewhat divergent ways of thinking about curing and healing. The well-defined definitions of these terms in *Black Belt Healing* go a long way to help dissipate the myths that surround hypnosis as well as other healing strategies involving the use of thought energy. Dr. Nelson has done quite well at bringing demystification, simplification, and utilization of the subject to an open, well-lit area.

This book does much more than present a method of pain management: this book creates an excellent new paradigm for living that includes a wide variety of guided and self-improvement strategies. A well-trained martial art instructor is in an excellent position to help students as well as non-students deal with some pain or achieve other goals that we have set before ourselves. Having said this, I would like to have you enjoy this particular journey as well as the many adventures that lie ahead as you move through *Black Belt Healing*.

Grandmaster Stacey A. Shook, PhD
Founder of Fu Chen Kung Fu

Introduction

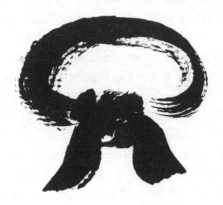

When martial artists ask me what I do for a living, I answer: "I teach people how to conquer pain."

Almost immediately I receive a "Really? How do you do that?" You see they want to know, because pain is a martial artist's constant companion and, at times, a nemesis.

I then briefly explain how the mind is a dojo…and contained in your Mind's Dojo are all the powerful weapons you need to win the war over pain. You simply need to learn the secrets of how to access them…and then use them correctly. I teach these secrets. I am a practitioner of Mind-Swords Hypnosis, and you can be too.

Black Belt Healing is based on my twenty-plus years of real-life clinical counseling experiences helping people cope naturally with pain and my own forty bruised and banged up years as a Karate-ka. Over these years, I have had the opportunity to work with many martial artists regarding martial, meditative, and healing arts. At my workshops, excited and interested participants have asked for written information about my hypnotic healing theories and pain management techniques. They want to continue to practice these pain management and healing arts at home for themselves…and perhaps to help loved ones as well.

You are holding the result of those inquiries.

Designed to be a practical how-to guide, you will discover how to use the power of your mind to not only conquer chronic pain, but to achieve a higher level of martial skill along with more inner peace and contentment as well. A tall order I know, and as you are reading this you are probably wondering if Mind-Swords Hypnosis can really help you. As most intelligent readers do, you may have already flipped through some of the pages, perhaps even checked the table of contents. I can assure you, what you will find will be transformative and eye opening.

My own recent experiences with a meniscus tear in my left knee once again validated the power of my mind in providing relief from pain and recovery from injury. While doing some heavy bag work I threw a series of roundhouse kicks. Upon completion my left knee felt a bit fuzzy and tingly. I didn't think much about it till later when my knee started to swell and ache. When I walked there was a clicking sensation. What bothered me the most about the knee was not being able to kneel down to bow in for Karate class or to sit cross-legged for meditation. The pain was too intense and I was very frustrated in not being able to do what I love to do. Even walking and doing daily chores like mowing my lawn eventually became more difficult and painful.

Incorporating a variety of visualizations and strategies you will be learning in this book, I was able to successfully manage the pain and over the course of three months able to sit in a kneeling position and cross my legs for meditation. The hypnotic technique I used that numbed my pain and helped me bend my knee into the position I desired was Te-Katana Anesthesia. After that, it has been great! I still can do heavy bag work with roundhouse kicks! More importantly, it validated my belief in the power of the mind.

It is important to note, however, this book is not a substitute for appropriate medical care, but rather, an adjunct healing art designed to facilitate recovery from pain. Pain of not only the body, but the mind and spirit as well. The art of Mind-Swords Hypnosis is grounded in scientifically proven methods of hypnosis as well as the time-honored principles and practices of Zen and Buddhist Psychology. They are safe and relevant for everyone, martial artist and non-martial artist alike.

As you explore the deep inner regions of your mind, body, and spirit with the philosophy and techniques in this book you will find more than just relief from pain and suffering. You will find a whole new way of viewing the world. Mind-Swords Hypnosis takes you there.

How this Book is Organized

This book is divided into three distinct parts.

Part One is designed to be your initial tour through your Mind's Dojo. Remember when you first went to your dojo to sign up for lessons? You were most likely given a tour and some history about the art, what it is used for, as well as your commitments such as showing up on time, keeping your uniform clean, and being respectful of others, right? This is what Part One will do for you. You will learn about your art, in this case Black Belt Healing, and be given a tour of your Mind's Dojo, along with the rules of conduct and how Mind-Swords Hypnosis can defend you against pain. Part One lays the foundation for your success. You will also learn some fast-acting pain relief hypnotic strategies.

Part Two begins your formal training in the Art of Mind-Swords Hypnosis. You will learn the How-to-Do of self-hypnosis and its relevant self-defense applications against the attack of pain. You will discover how it is just like going to the Dojo to work out with some really cool swords. I kid you not.

Part Three is your Catalog of Techniques to Mind-Swords Hypnosis mastery. It guides you step-by-step with hypnotic scripts and strategies designed exclusively for the martial artist. These are the actual Samurai-like Mind-Sword techniques you will use to conquer pain and transform your life!

Starting with Chapter 1, each chapter builds on the previous one, providing you with the opportunity to continually reinforce what you have learned. You will go through the natural progression of what it takes to enter the gate of your Mind's Dojo, the subconscious mind, use your Mind-Swords and transform yourself. It's like having your own personal tour guide walking you hand in hand through the entire process.

You will also notice I have included a variety of Zen stories I learned from my Zen teacher, Nonin, and various Zen stories and koans I have learned over the years. As you may be aware, koans are Zen riddles or stories that create "space in your mind," confusion, or a state of bewilderment. When the mind is struck with awe or confusion, it is more open to insight and, more importantly, change.

The old Zen Masters knew this and used koans to help their students break the conditioning of their minds and see into their true nature. These koans benefit you in the same way. They will hopefully help you remember to create that open space of mind within yourself as you learn.

How to Use This Book

Black Belt Healing will take you step-by-step through the process of managing and healing pain with hypnosis and hypnosis-related healing arts. You will learn how to practice hypnosis for your own benefit and learn how to help others, perhaps family members, students or lay people…if you choose to do so.

During each step you will learn valuable mind/body principles of healing that will change the way you view and respond to pain. While reading and learning the material, I encourage you to take notes. As you read the material, thoughts and ideas will pop into your mind on how you can personally apply these principles and steps to your life and the lives of others. When this happens, write the ideas down. It's possible that many ideas will come to you and you can refer to these notes as you develop your hypnotherapy skills and healing abilities.

There is a wealth of information contained in this course and my advice is to go through the entire book, then go through it again, but more mindfully. This will help with your learning and retention. Then, more importantly, begin to apply the steps. Just reading the book and thinking you know how to do hypnosis is like reading a book on jujutsu and thinking you know how to defend yourself. You only truly know it when you do it. Wouldn't you agree?

And, as you are aware, nearly anyone can quickly and easily learn some basic self-defense skills and feel more confident, but it does not make them a black belt. The same goes for hypnosis: practice is essential.

Important Skills and Facts You Will Learn From This Book.

Here they are. You will learn:
1. How to get pain relief fast.
2. How to hypnotize yourself quickly and easily.
3. How to conquer pain with mind power.
4. How to plant post-hypnotic suggestions for continuous healing.
5. How to hypnotize family and friends for health and healing.
6. How to realistically manage the emotional suffering that comes with pain.
7. How your mind is a dojo with weapons of healing.
8. How hypnosis is shrouded in myth and misconception.
9. How to apply martial strategies to heal pain.
10. How to use street-effective pain management techniques.
11. How to gain quick access to your subconscious mind.
12. How to use your Mind-Swords for pain relief.
13. How to enter the "secret" gate to gain access to pure raw healing potential.
14. How to use your Mind-Swords to give you life.

15. How to win the three battles that come with pain.
16. How to not feed the bears.
17. How to practice authentic Zen meditation.
18. How to activate your natural healing defenses.
19. The truth about hypnosis certification.
20. The true healing meaning of "Budo."
21. How to keep hypnosis legal if you decide to help family or
    friends.

Terminology

A majority of the martial art terms used in this book come from my experience in the Okinawan/Japanese traditions. Translations of the terms will appear in parentheses throughout the book.

Part One

When you meet someone attained in the Tao
on the road, do not make your greeting with words
or with silence.

How will you make your greeting?

CHAPTER 1

The Paradox of Pain

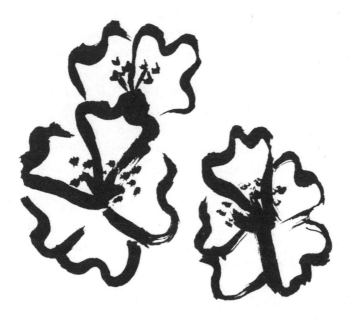

Imagine for a moment what it would be like if you could earn a Black Belt without pain? It wouldn't be so special now would it? As you are aware, the path to a black belt is paved with pain. Pain is the relentless sensei who gives you no rest, no slack, no mercy, no escape. Pain is the dojo-mate who breaks your ribs and bloodies your nose. Pain is the sore back and shoulder you receive from being slam-dunked into the mat…over and over. I am sure you will agree with me, if you want to master your art, you must look deeply into yourself, and come to grips with your pain.

Most of us easily handle the usual and expected pain of training. Typically, this type of pain subsides within a brief period of time. A little aspirin, ointment, or the Chinese healing liniment, Dit Da Jow, along with some rest, and you are up and back in the dojo within days or a few weeks. But what about the pain that lingers?

What about the pain that stays with you months after the insult or injury has subsided and you are now feeling edgy and frustrated? What about the pain that causes you to lose sleep, not for days, but for weeks on end? What about the nagging pain the martial artist has after decades of practice? In these pages you will learn how to manage this type of pain.

There is something primal about pain. It is adrenaline pumping and mind focusing. As a martial artist you might welcome the pain of being the recipient of a well placed arm-bar for learning or demonstration purposes; however, that is vastly different from the unwelcome pain of being the recipient of a not-so-well executed arm-bar by an inexperienced student.

In this chapter, and those to follow, you will learn more about pain and its primal nature. You will learn its habits and how to successfully manage those habits. Think about it this way. Just like fighting an opponent in the ring, it is usually important to know as much about him or her so you can prepare your strategy. This is what you are going to do for your opponent of pain. So, your first step is to study and learn about the different types of pain and how to identify them. Consider this your pre-fight strategy meeting.

Now, I am not going to get into the biology, chemistry or neurology of pain. One thing we all know is that when we are in pain we want it to stop. We want relief…and we want relief yesterday. There is, however, some merit in understanding the anatomy of pain, but it is such a wide subject that I tend to do the Zen thing and keep it simple.

There are basically two types of pain: Acute and Chronic. Acute pain is the pain you experience immediately after an accident, like a punch to the ribs, or onset of an illness, like the flu. The rule of thumb is it generally lasts less than six months; after that it is considered chronic. Fortunately, both chronic and acute pain respond equally well to Black Belt Healing.

Now, let's examine pain more closely for a moment. As you will notice it is actually a very broad descriptor for a myriad of uncomfortable physical sensations in the body. When you are experiencing pain, trying to run from it or fight it does not really help you all that much. Recall that you must know your enemy very well. This entails becoming knowledgeable about it and labeling it.

Consider this for a moment. If you wanted to help someone in pain, being told she or he has pain really does not tell you anything especially useful does it? It is like hearing someone telling you they practiced kata for an hour and need some help with the bunkai (application of movement). Kata is a broad label for a countless number of physical movements within the art of Karate. To truly be helpful, the student needs to be specific about which kata and which movement. Was it Sanchin, Naihanchi, and/or Seisan? Then you can be helpful and go into specifics.

The same goes for your own pain. If you were to "get in the ring" with pain you want to know what it is, what its background is, how much it weighs, what is its reach. Just like your opponents come in many shapes and sizes, pain comes in a countless number of forms. Besides being acute or chronic, it can be called general, specific, referred, phantom, occasional, constant, physical, emotional, psychological, even spiritual in nature. It can be described as stabbing, gripping, burning, shooting, dull aching, sharp, throbbing, cutting, pinching, twisting, penetrating, heavy, cutting, drilling, freezing, hot, racing, squeezing, splitting, etc. I think you get the picture.

These descriptors are important as they help you identify the mindset and imagery you are using. Words like "throbbing, "stabbing," and "exploding" brings up images of a dynamic, moving, and active pain. Words like "aching," or "tooth ache numb" imply a more static, lingering type of pain. Regardless of the descriptor images, they will help guide you into the type of Mind-Sword Hypnosis technique you are going to use against it.

For instance, David, a Judo practitioner, tore his left rotator cuff (he actually hurt himself on the job) and eventually had surgery to repair it. After surgery he still had a *searing, red hot* pain radiating throughout his shoulder. He also discussed the amount of *anger* he had over the work injury and how he was treated…he was let go for not being able to do his job as a carpenter. Despite the pain, his doctor gave him a release. David came to see me about one year after the surgery. He was depressed, had difficulty sleeping, and constantly felt on–edge.

These descriptors allowed me to develop a healing strategy for David. Listening to his descriptors and story, sessions were designed to elicit pictures of a blue, cooling anesthetic in the form of a special ointment similar to Dit Da Jow. He was familiar with the Chinese liniment Dit Da Jow and had a deep belief in its healing elements. He left the sessions feeling better and amazed how his mind could influence his pain perceptions.

At this point in time, I want you to get a piece of paper and a pen or pencil. I want you to do a little exercise and write down your current type of pain. Is it acute or chronic? Then begin to list descriptors. Is it hot or cold? Throbbing or pounding? How would you label it?

On a scale of 0-10, with 10 being the most intense pain you can tolerate, what number are you? You would be surprised how many people find it difficult to label their pain as they are not really in tune with their bodies. I am sure you will do fine, but just in case here is a simple way to get in touch with your pain. I call it the "But" or "If only" techniques.

With your pencil write out, "My discomfort does not bother me… but," (then write down the first "buts" that come to mind. Then write, "My discomfort does not bother me throughout the day, except…" Then write down your "excepts." Next write, "My discomfort does not bother me at all, if only…" then write down your "if onlys." Again, write down the first thoughts that come to your mind. Don't over think the process just let it flow. Keep this list. You will need it later.

A journey of a thousand miles begins with the first step.

Which foot do you start with?

CHAPTER 2

The Saimon-jutsu Solution

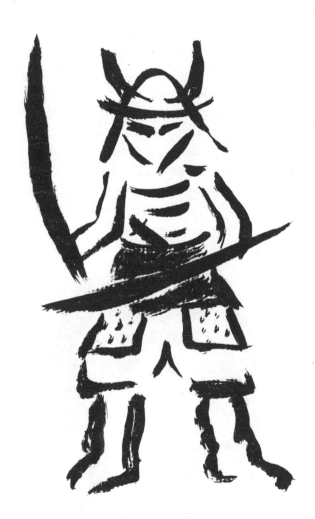

"You are getting sleepy…your eyelids are getting heavy now…and as I now count from 10 to 1 you will find yourself drifting down, down, down into hypnosis…you are feeling so safe and secure now…"

This is probably the image you have of someone going into hypnosis…and you are partially right. Have you ever been so engrossed in a Bruce Lee movie that you felt you were part of the action? Or have perhaps driven to the dojo, getting there, but not remembering how you got there? Or gotten so lost in a daydream that you could see and feel everything as if it were real? This is your mind lost in trance. You were hypnotized!

Hypnosis has been around for centuries and most cultures have some form of its practice. The Japanese term for hypnosis is *Saimon-jutsu*. It comes from the Chinese term, *Hsi Men Jitsu*, which means, "techniques for opening the mind's gate."

This is exactly what you are doing when you are practicing hypnosis. Hypnosis is the key that allows you to unlock and enter your Mind's Gate in order to reach the deep subconscious. It is used worldwide to help people make positive health changes, such as losing weight, stopping smoking or quitting other habits, such as nail-biting. It is also used in the medical profession for stress and pain management.

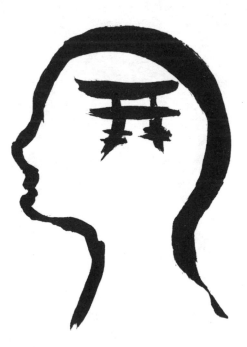

Mind's Gate

Hypnosis is also a healing art that uses your mind's natural ability to drift, float, and daydream. During this day-dreamy state your powerful subconscious mind is very sensitive and open to positive suggestion. As you will soon learn, the subconscious mind is responsible for deep and lasting change as well as physical perception. Yes, physical perception. Anything can seem possible. So, if you can daydream, you can be hypnotized. You can conquer pain!

Myths and Frequently Asked Questions About Hypnosis

Hypnosis, just like the martial arts, is often shrouded in myth and misconception. Remember a moment when someone unfamiliar with the martial arts found out you practiced a martial art? What was their reaction? If your experiences were like mine, their perception of what you do was way off the mark, if not downright embarrassing.

Just think of all the crazy ideas people have of you when you tell them you practice karate, jujutsu, or kung fu.

The same goes for hypnosis. The general public's impression of hypnosis comes from watching television or watching a stage hypnotist make a fool out of people. Because hypnosis has been masked in mystery and misunderstanding, some people are afraid of using it. Their irrational fears include being forced to "cluck like a chicken" or doing some other silly thing they've witnessed from stage hypnotists. Some people are even concerned I am going to take control of their mind for evil purposes...I kid you not.

In case you were wondering how safe hypnosis is, it has been approved and sanctioned by the American Medical Association since 1958. When you seriously look at it, all methods of hypnosis are actually a form of self-hypnosis. Even with a trained hypnotherapist guiding you through the process, *you must be willing to let it happen.* Without your complete and total willingness to participate and receive the suggestions, hypnosis will not occur. It simply will not happen.

It's a fact: Hypnosis is no more dangerous than daydreaming. You can't get forever stuck in hypnosis any more than you can get forever stuck in an idle daydream. (Of course, we all have had those daydreams we *wish* we could get stuck in. But it just can't happen.) So, if you can daydream, you can do hypnosis. Hypnosis is simply therapeutic daydreaming.

Just think how fast you snapped out of a daydream when your fifth grade teacher called your name in the middle of a math lesson. The same happens with hypnosis. If during a hypnosis session you were in a deep trance and a fire alarm went off, you would respond quickly and appropriately with no ill effects.

Here are some of the most frequently asked questions about hypnosis:

Can I be controlled under hypnosis?

No. Under hypnosis you would not do anything that you normally wouldn't do. You are NOT under the control of the hypnotist. No one can be hypnotized against his or her will.

Can I get stuck in hypnosis?

No. No one can get stuck in hypnosis. All you have to do is open your eyes and end the trance. It's that simple. You are always, and I repeat, *always* in control.

Who can be hypnotized?

Almost anyone can be hypnotized. In fact, you hypnotize yourself many times a day, but you call it daydreaming or mind-wandering. For instance, have you ever had the experience of driving to a familiar place but accidently bypass the correct exit? You were hypnotized.

Will I be able to go into a hypnotic state?

Motivation is the key to entering into hypnosis. You must be a willing partner. All you have to do is listen and cooperate.

Will I have difficulty awakening?

No. Again, you are in total control and can end the session anytime you desire.

So, you may be wondering just about now, "What is the difference between regular hypnosis and Mind-Sword Hypnosis?" This is a very good question. First, Mind-Sword Hypnosis is a method of healing that employs a model of mind you won't find anywhere else. Secondly, Mind-Sword Hypnosis has a focus more similar to a martial art than a healing art. Mind-Sword Hypnosis and martial arts are both systems of self-defense. "Goshin," or self-preservation, is their mutual and common goal.

Think about this for a moment. Whether you are attacked by an assailant carrying a knife or whether the stabbing pain of arthritis is attacking you, you are being attacked. Therefore, a system of "self-defense" is needed in either scenario. When your arthritis pain stabs you, Mind-Sword Hypnosis supplies the appropriate techniques to counteract that pain.

By the same token, both martial arts systems and the Mind-Sword Hypnosis system have foundational techniques (Kihon Waza) to learn, practice, and master…and both are designed to make you feel safe, secure, and protected from pain. As a seasoned martial artist, you already possess a framework of defense principles and practice. You know the human anatomy and even some basic psychology. So, who is better equipped than you, a martial artist, to understand the principles of Mind-Sword Hypnosis as a self-defense system and help yourself and, perhaps others, defend themselves from the attack of pain?

We have already established the fact that you face pain every time you step onto the dojo floor and in many cases you take it home with you and to work. Just as effectiveness on the street is the measure of any good martial art, so must it be with a healing art. Mind-Sword Hypnosis is such an art. It is not only effective, but, as you will see, extremely "street savvy."

But what about Mary?

The student asked the master, "What is Buddha?"

The master replied, "This mind is Buddha."

CHAPTER 3

What About Mary?

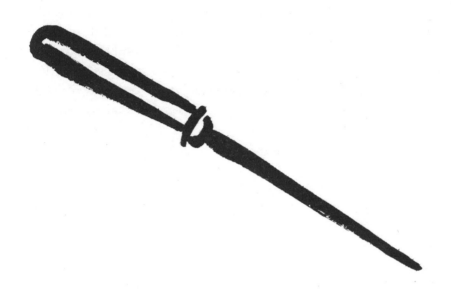

Mary was a slender 5'11" woman in her early 30's. She came to see me to because she had pain from arthritis in her lower spine. She described it as a solid, steel ice pick stuck in her lower back. The sensation rarely subsided, and it caused her turmoil at home and at work. Her goal was to feel less pain, achieve more calmness throughout the day and to feel like she was in control of her life again.

Her sessions with me included some lessons in Qigong, visualizations of healing, along with a variety of hypnosis sessions designed to move her Qi and "see" herself as being well. Because her brother was a Kung Fu practitioner Mary was familiar with the martial arts. She told him what she was doing and my background:

He told her to listen and trust me. She's glad she did. After one month of Mind-Sword Hypnosis she began to report feeling more relaxed and in control, even though her pain levels were still present.

Mary eventually learned how to relax *into* her pain with a variety of guided visualizations and to develop a sense of curiosity about her pain rather than trying to fight it. She also instituted a daily meditation routine of just being present with her pain. Three months later she came to tell me, with a smile reaching from ear to ear: her ice pick had disappeared! It had lost its sharpness and turned into a "scrubby piece of steel wool." Obviously, Mary found this experience much more to her liking, but what is really noteworthy is her arthritis was still there. It had not gone away. Mary had received a *healing*, but her back was not *cured*. How is this possible? Let's take a look.

Healing Versus Curing

A cure occurs when a treatment or series of treatments removes all evidence of the disease that is causing the pain. This allows a person, like Mary, to live as comfortably as she would without arthritis. Curing is typically an application of an external medical process, like surgery or medicines. These influence a biological or chemical change that causes the disease to disappear. Think of it as a well-placed straight punch to an opponent's nose. It is hard, or yang, in nature and attempts to knock out the discomfort directly. In this example, the biological change is your opponent now lying face down on the floor. Your "dis-ease" has been removed.

Healing also involves a treatment or series of treatments, but rather working solely on a biological or chemical level, it provides relief more holistically. Healing incorporates the use of your entire being: the body, mind, emotions, energy (Qi or Ki), and spirit. Rather than remove all evidence of disease directly, healing treatments stimulate your body's natural defenses to provide relief. Healing harmonizes with the disease just like a good Aikido-ka harmonizes with an attack before slamming you into the earth. The healing treatments are more yin, softer and yielding, yet very effective. You were born with a natural defense system against discomfort and disease. Healing simply enhances this innate wisdom.

As you examine this more closely, healing goes beyond what curing can provide. Healing typically involves a holistic mind-expansive paradigm-shaking emotional transformation along with physical relief. Why? Because, as you will see, holism (seeing a bigger picture) and emotions lie in your Mind's Dojo, the subconscious mind. This is where deep and lasting change occurs for your safety and protection. It is important to note that, just like Mary, healing can take place even when curing is not possible. Mary's perception and relationship to her pain changed on a very deep and intimate level that goes beyond biology. This transformation gave Mary a shift of perspective, an inner sense of control, and an ability to act with greater balance and security.

Just like learning a new self-defense skill, healing makes you feel more balanced and secure. In many respects, your martial art is a healing art. You have been given new ways of seeing yourself as you have been challenged to find inner resources you never knew you had. This in turn provides you with a greater sense of confidence, balance, control, and security. Mind-Sword Hypnosis is considered a healing art, not a curing art. Please take note of this.

Now let's take a tour of your mind.

If you take off both wheels and the axle of a cart,
what would be vividly apparent?

CHAPTER 4
Kokoro Kobe Dojo

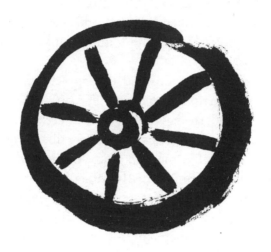

Wouldn't it be amazing if you had a map to the mind that revealed to you the intricate details of how to effectively heal pain and constructively manage your life? Well, you are about to find one. You see, a few years ago while helping a young woman manage the suffering she had from fibromyalgia, an idea hit me like a roundhouse kick to the head! My mind is a dojo!

I could see how the floor plan of a Japanese dojo is a map to the mind and personal power. It became suddenly clear to me that in my Mind's Dojo, the subconscious mind, are all the weapons I needed to battle pain and facilitate healing. I was, to say the least, very excited! And when you see how it can help you, you will be too.

What makes Mind-Sword Hypnosis different from other styles of hypnosis is this model of the mind. There is an old Zen saying that goes like this, "*Kokoro Kobe Dojo.*" It translates to "*Your Mind is Your*

Dojo." As you may be aware, a dojo is a place where you physically train in your art, but it is also where you intimately investigate the spiritual and sacred aspects of your life.

The word "dojo" is comprised of two Chinese characters. The first is do or "Way" and, secondly, jo or "Place." Literally, it is where you practice "The Way." This "Way" alludes to being in harmony with the universal energy known as Tao (Dow) and is reflected in the "-do" after martial arts such as kendo, karate-do, tae kwon do, aikido or judo. "*Kokoro Kobe Dojo*" forms the foundation and is the model for Black Belt Healing.

When you examine a traditional dojo practicing Japanese budo (the Way of the Warrior....hey, another -do) you will find some similarities with modern-day dojo's with one exception. Have you ever noticed how modern dojos look more like fitness centers or dance studios? Well, unlike modern dojo's, traditional dojo's have the feel, smell, and look of a Shinto or Buddhist temple. A *Kamidana*, or altar/shrine, is present and is a focal point to remind the practitioners of the sacredness and spirit of their practice. The dojo then becomes a special and sacred space, where not only is your character is perfected through arduous training, but spiritual enlightenment is cultivated and nurtured. My Sensei often reminded us that dojo means "Hall of Enlightenment."

I grew up in the Midwest and when you visit someone's home for the first time you usually were invited for a quick tour. So, that's what I am going to do now. I am going to give you a quick look-see into your mind as modeled by a traditional Japanese dojo. Subsequent chapters will go into further detail.

Welcome to my home...and yours as well. When you first enter from the street, the room you encounter is the *Genkan*, or foyer. This is where you place your street clothes and shoes and perhaps change into your workout uniform or "gi." It may be decorated with diplomas, pictures or scrolls. It is usually a small space.

As you can see in the diagram, separating the genkan and formal dojo is the "*mon*," or gate. This is where you bow prior to entering the formal training room, the dojo. This mon is usually at the "foot" of the dojo. After bowing, you enter the dojo and avail yourself of the workout equipment and weapons. You also spend some time in meditation in front of the Kamidana or altar, usually situated at the "head" of the dojo.

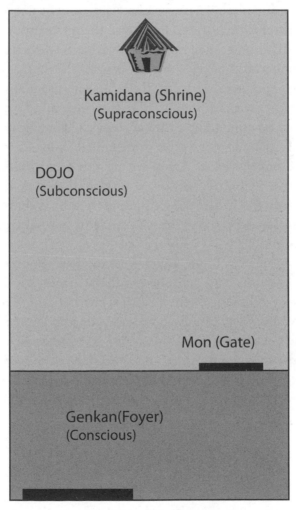

Kokoro Kobe Dojo

As you tour the dojo, or your mind in this case, you will notice, like most rooms, genkans, mons, dojo's and Kamidana's have three distinct features. First, they have a purpose. For instance, your kitchen's purpose is to store and prepare food. Secondly, rooms are furnished to fulfill the room's purpose. Your kitchen typically comes complete with a stove, refrigerator, cupboards, table and sink so you can store food, cook it, and wash up afterwards. And, last but not least, rooms have rules. Kitchen rules could be to shut the refrigerator door when done, turn off burners when not in use, wash your dishes after eating, and, most importantly, keep the cook happy.

Since the dojo is modeled after the mind, let's use it as a map. Your mind also has two main "rooms", the conscious mind (genkan) and the subconscious mind (dojo). They are separated by a "gate" called the discriminating mind (mon), or in professional hypnosis, it is referred to as the "Critical Factor." Deep within the subconscious mind is another gate (symbolized by the Kamidana), that connects more intimately with the Tao, or sometimes referred to as supraconscious, universal consciousness, or spiritual source of our being. This is my favorite room.

Each room of your mind, along with its dojo counterpart, has a functional purpose. It is decorated with furnishings and has rules of behavior or etiquette. In the next few chapters you will learn the strong correlation between the dojo and your mind. Revealed to you will be the Conscious, Discriminating, and Subconscious Mind's purpose, how they are furnished and the rules to follow to be able to maximize their abilities and help you heal yourself. You will also learn about the Supraconscious Mind, which makes all creation of healing possible.

Two monks were arguing about the temple flag waving in the wind. One said, "The flag moves." The other said, "The wind moves." They argued back and forth but could not agree.

The old master said, "Gentlemen. It is not the wind that moves; it is not the flag that moves; it is your mind that moves."

CHAPTER 5

The Genkan –
Your Conscious Mind

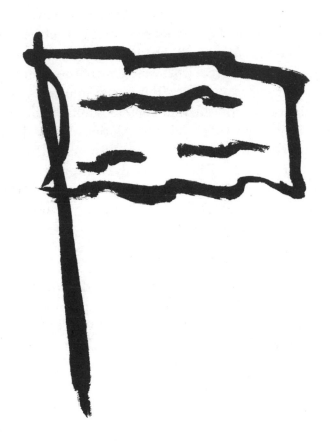

As you have learned, before you can enter the formal training hall to practice your art, you must enter the genkan, or foyer. It lies outside the formal training hall, or the dojo. Correspondingly, your conscious mind is considered the genkan of your mind and lies just outside your Mind's Dojo or the subconscious mind. Let's examine the genkan/conscious mind in more detail.

Furnishings: As you walk through the genkan you see it is furnished with a shoe rack to place your shoes and might also have pictures of accomplishments or certificates of rank on the wall. In modern times, a changing room can also be considered a genkan and furnished with hooks, lockers, or showers.

Consequently, prior to entering your Mind's Dojo, you must start in your Mind's Genkan, the conscious mind. It is furnished with your six senses of taste, touch, smell, hearing, sight, and consciousness. Together, these form the "you" when you think of your self. This is your Ego. This is your sense of identity. This is your mind that moves.

As you might have noticed, your conscious mind is also furnished with the ability to provide workable solutions as to "how things work." This part of your mind is supplied with a wonderful computer-like ability to categorize, label, and analyze in order to solve your day-to-day problems. As you probably have deduced, this is the realm of your logical reasoning. Here's where you use and gather information; access short-term memory; and apply logic using words, numbers, facts, and figures. This is where you spend most of your waking time.

Another, and very important, furnishing of the conscious mind is your willpower. Your willpower is an integral part of the conscious mind. Believe it or not, it is a combination of your ego-identity, free will, and intentions. You tend to use it after you have logically solved a problem and then try to effect positive behavioral change. This could be to eat fewer sweets, if you are overweight, or learning a new kata for the next belt promotion, or keeping with the focus of this book.

The problem with willpower is that it is intimately connected to your ego and thinks it is an independent agent that doesn't need any help. If you know any egocentric people, you know what I am talking about. As you will read later, willpower becomes much more effective when it teams up with the part of the subconscious mind that is actually responsible for changing habits and inducing authentic and transformational healings.

Purpose: The purpose of the genkan is to store your shoes and clothes prior to entering the dojo for formal training. This is where you leave behind your worldly ideas, intellectualization, ego, and personal identity. You are no longer a butcher, baker, or candlestick maker, but a student of the "Way."

The primary purpose of the conscious mind, if you haven't figured it out by now, is to store your "shoes" or ego, and to logically solve problems. Once solved intellectually, then willpower is used in an attempt to make the necessary changes.

Rules: In the genkan, the rules provide order. Here your shoes must be aligned properly, heels to the wall, toes pointing outward. Your gi must be clean and white, obi tied appropriately and you are to prepare yourself for training. Talking is kept to a minimum.

In order to give you optimum use of your conscious mind's functions and furnishings certain rules must be followed. There are basically three of them:

Rule One: Be alert and oriented. A conscious mind that is asleep is not conscious!

Rule Two: Use input from the six senses, then gather and assimilate the information by processing words, numbers, facts, and figures.

Rule Three: Navigate intention and willpower in positive directions. This is good for short-term change and provides the impetus for the beginning of change.

Following these rules will give you the best use of your conscious mind. Just like in your home it is easier to cook food in the kitchen because that is where the stove, fridge, pots, pans, and food are located. It is easier to analyze problems with the conscious mind because that is where your alertness, intentions, logical reasoning, and willpower are located.

Lily is a good example of how to use your conscious mind. Lily suffered from the pain of fibromyalgia. One day while waiting for one of my appointments, Lily called me and wanted to know if she could come in later that day. She was having a very stressful time at work and her pain levels were high, so she was looking for some relief. Lily, was consciously aware of her situation, had reviewed her options, navigated her intention, and used her willpower to call me for an appointment. She was glad she did, because later that day she was able to de-stress and find the relief she was seeking.

In a nutshell, this is how to use your Mind's Genkan, the conscious mind. It is who you are prior to entering the subconscious to effect change. Before you can enter your Mind's Dojo for training you must open and pass through the Mind's Gate.

But there is a small problem.

Show me now, how do you open the gateless gate?

CHAPTER 6
Enter the Gate

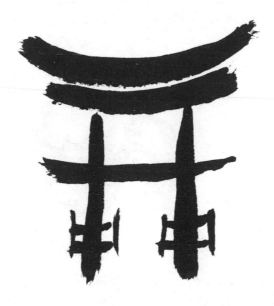

As you read earlier, the Japanese term for hypnosis is Saimon-jutsu or "Techniques for Opening the Mind's Gate." The entrance to the dojo is very important as it provides access to the training hall, your dojo. However, as I mentioned, there is a problem: The mon has a guardian.

Furnishings: Have you ever seen a Fu Dog or Chinese Lion? These are those funny looking animals that are a hybrid of a dog and a lion. They are usually seen outside the entrance to Buddhist temples. They are guardians of the gates and designed to scare away intruders.

Your Mind's Gate is also furnished with its own version of a Fu Dog. It is called discrimination and in the profession of hypnosis it is called the Critical Factor because it is the part that critiques.

Discrimination judges information that comes to the gate, either from the conscious side or the subconscious. Here is what this guard does:

Purpose One: Maintain the Status Quo of the Ego. It does this by filtering ideas and information that arise from the subconscious to the conscious. The guardian of your gate strives to keep information that comes up from the subconscious in line with your perception of self.

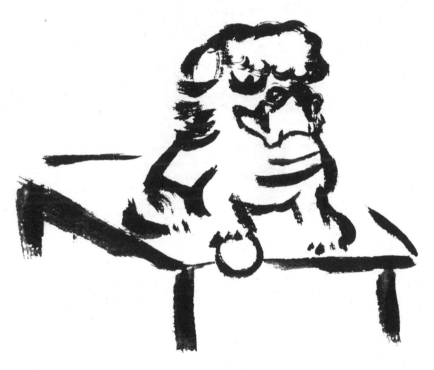

Fu Dog/Chinese Lion

It discriminates whether a certain idea or image fits your personal construct of how you think you and reality should be. You can say this part of your mind also holds your self-limiting beliefs. Its purpose is to help your conscious mind keep and make sense of your self and the world. If too much information floods your conscious mind it gets overloaded with sensory information, possibly resulting in a nervous breakdown—which is not something you want to experience.

Purpose Two: Protects the Subconscious Mind From Change. The gate acts as a veil over the subconscious to keep it from being invaded. The role of the guardian is to keep you from accessing the subconscious mind too deeply to activate change. As you will learn, the subconscious mind is protective, a bit lazy, and does not like change. It wants to keep intruders out, especially intruders like your ego and willpower.

Have you ever had the experience of recognizing someone while walking down the street, but can't recall their name? You know their face, perhaps where they work or live, but can't find the name? The harder your willpower tries to access the long term memory bank located in the subconscious mind, the Fu Dog at the gate is doing his job and blocks entry. You are trying to get in without permission and you are not allowed access. The forceful, ego-centered attempt of willpower to access your subconscious is denied because it is not following the rules.

The Rules.

There are two rules to abide by in order to pass the guardian of the gate:

Rule One:
Suspend your sense of self by adopting shoshin (beginner's mind).
Remember the stories of old when a student wished to study with a certain master he had to humble himself with menial chores and subservience? This was a testing period to determine the prospective student's willingness to train diligently with an open mind and honest intentions. Even in zen training, a prospective monk must wait outside the temple gate for at least three days (or more) prior to formal entrance.

In more modern times, putting on a white gi (uniform) symbolizes this willingness to have an open mind to train, change, and grow. Despite your social standing outside the dojo, whether you are a physician, lawyer, dishwasher, student, or unemployed, you are all equal on the inside of the dojo. This is leaving your ego in the genkan.

Standing at the entrance of the gate, a formal bow is necessary - this represents shoshin. This bow prepares the mind and spirit for the transformation about to take place once you enter the dojo floor. Adopting shoshin and bowing, you allow yourself to be open to change. This is the "password" speak that the Fu Dog recognizes. This enables you to pass through the gate and communicate directly with your subconscious mind.

Rule Two:
When bowing at the gate also have an attitude of gratitude.
Be thankful for the opportunity to train in the dojo of your mind. Gratitude keeps your mind's gate open and receptive to change, especially in the face of discouragement and despair. Sometimes pain does not disappear as fast as you want it to, but if you remain grateful, even for the pain, healing occurs.

The act of bowing embodies, not only shoshin, but a grateful mind. Beginner's mind and grateful mind are like two sides of the same coin. Together they form an embodiment of enlightenment. This might sound weird, but begin bowing with a great depth of gratitude to all things, animate and inanimate, and notice the changes that begin to happen. One of my enlightening and healing moments came to me when I witnessed Nonin, my Zen teacher, bowing in deep respect to a toilet! (And no, he didn't have a lot of Japanese beer the night before). Bow often.

The world is vast and wide.

Why do you wear your sword when you bow into the training hall?

CHAPTER 7

Your Mind's Dojo

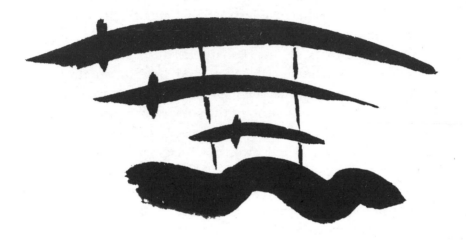

This is probably one of the most important and longest chapters of the book. It contains a wealth of information, as the dojo of your mind is vast. You will do yourself a favor by reading this carefully and then re-reading it.

Furnishings: Continuing our tour, after bowing, and passing the guardian of the gate, you enter into the formal training hall, the dojo. A traditional dojo is a wide open space furnished with training gear such as weights, punching bags, mats, and makiwara boards. Also included are weapons such as bokken, bo, jo, sai, kama, and swords. Last but not least is the Kamidana, or altar. Once inside the dojo you can now avail yourself of the furnishings to conduct your training.

Your subconscious mind, your Mind's Dojo, also has many furnishings. It is primarily furnished with the Katana (long sword) of Imagery, the Wakazashi (short sword) of Emotions and the Tanto (knife) of Faith. These are your three powerful Mind-Swords.

Take note. As you begin to use your Mind-Swords it is of the utmost importance that you know how to use them. They are as sharp as real swords and if not used properly can cause untold damage. Imagine for a moment handing a razor-sharp katana to an untrained novice and tell him to practice swinging the sword and sheathing it, but without providing real instruction. Odds are he will cut off a finger, thumb, or toe along the way.

Our Mind-Swords are just as sharp. If left to the untrained, like the imagination running wild, it can do more harm than good. Remember a moment when perhaps as a child, you were called to the principal's office or as an adult the boss wants to see you. What's the first thing that popped into your head? Yeah, you thought you were in trouble. Your Mind-Sword of Imagination can cut you. If left unchecked, it can actually kill you! When trained properly in its use, however, Mind-Swords can heal and transform your life.

Your subconscious mind also contains training tools. These are your long-term memories: the good, the bad, and the ugly. Yes, they are all there, stored and ready for your use. Another training tool is your ingrained auto-pilot habits. This makes training easier, like using mats for falling. Auto-pilot kicks in to make tying your obi (belt) easier or remembering a kata. Your subconscious is also the repository for your Karmic Seeds. Karmic Seeds are the results of your actions, both from this life and past lives as well as the seeds of potential.

You might find this interesting. Deep within your subconscious is another gate. This gate is the entrance to the spiritual part of your self. It has also been called the Great Void, Emptiness, Tao, supraconscious, collective unconscious, or Allaya consciousness. This is the true source of what I like to call "Raw Pure Potential."

The Kamidana (altar or shrine) in traditional dojos reflect this connection to the greater spiritual part of our self. It is a very important part of a traditional dojo's furnishings. I will touch more upon this in a later chapter.

Purpose: The primary purpose of the dojo is training and transformation, both on a physical and spiritual level. It is here you train in the armed and unarmed arts for self-preservation. Did you know a formal dojo's layout is also designed for protection of the head instructor, the sensei or shihan? His or her seat is located in front of the Kamidana, opposite the entrance. If intruders were to break in, he would have good visibility and the intruders would have to get through the strategically positioned students.

So, guess what? The primary purpose of the subconscious mind is also transformative and protective. Your subconscious wants you to be whole and well, however, it does not have the problem solving skills of the conscious mind to determine what exactly is good or bad for you. In many ways it is like a two-year-old child that does not have the awareness or experience of what is good or bad. In this respect we need to train our subconscious properly or it will become dysfunctional.

The subconscious mind has three primary functions that help protect you:

Function One: Resist change. Remember the old joke that the only person who likes change is a wet baby? The same goes for your subconscious mind. It does not like to make changes. It likes its well-worn ruts, but again this is for your security. Basically, this is to keep all of your habits, emotions, and memory in a state of a balance and provide a sense of comfort. Change is kept slow as a self-protective function. Unfortunately, if you have trained your subconscious mind to accept that cigarettes help you relax, this resistance to change can actually hurt you. Why? Well, the longer an idea remains in the subconscious mind, the greater the opposition to change will occur and, as we all know, cigarette smoking causes cancer.

Let's examine this for a moment. Take for instance someone who has tried to quit smoking cigarettes after smoking for 15 or 20 years. The cigarettes give this smoker a sense of anxiety reduction, which the subconscious mind interprets this as good. Therefore, the subconscious keeps this person smoking regardless of what the willpower has decided through logical conclusions. The harder this person tries to quit the more the subconscious resists and makes quitting harder. Take note, in a battle between the subconscious mind and the conscious mind, the subconscious mind will always win...always. It is bigger and stronger.

Do you see how it works now? Every idea that enters the subconscious mind gets tested for safety and protection against what it has been programmed to believe is safe and good for you. It wants you to feel secure.

Function Two: Reflect and create a physical reaction based on what is "seen," whether what is "seen" is real or imagined. Just like a punch, slap, or kick causes a physical reaction in your opponent, so does every thought or sensory image you have causes a physical reaction. This is a key element. The body, mind, and spirit are all parts of a single entity and all phenomena are interconnected. If there is a change at any level of existence, it will affect all others, just like lined-up dominoes.

As you can probably gather by now, your thoughts and images influence all functions of your body. This is so important I am going to repeat it. *Your thoughts and images influence all functions of your body.* For instance, the thought and image of a lemon begins the salivation process. The thought and image of head lice brings scalp itching. The thought and image of going to a job you hate brings ulcers. The thought and image of a blue monkey brings a chuckle... did I mention he has a big red butt?

Couple this with resisting change, can you see now how once an idea is allowed and accepted into the subconscious mind, it will continue to produce the same physical reaction, over and over, until the idea is changed? So, to produce the physical action of healing, let's say, on a torn medial meniscus, image the meniscus healing itself or already healed. After I tore my left medial meniscus a few years ago and I pictured the meniscus sewn together and I would also mentally "iron" the meniscus, taking out the wrinkles and melting the tear.

These thoughts and images were delivered with strong emotions (which you will be learning how to do) of calm and success, teaching my subconscious mind that is okay to heal the meniscus. It worked.

Function Three: Create autopilot habits. This is to help make your life easier and, hopefully, more efficient. Your autonomic habits, like driving a car or tying your shoes makes life easier because you don't have to engage the conscious mind in analyzing the situation to do it.

Generally speaking, a mental auto-pilot habit is easier to perform than a conscious action. But once the conscious action becomes habit with repetition it will happen almost automatically. Remember as a child, trying to tie your shoes? It felt like one big arduous conscious step-by-step task, didn't it? Now, with frequent repetition, it is such an insignificant effort that you barely pay it any attention. Think of the first self-defense technique you ever learned, how difficult was it at first? With time, however, it's so simple.

Rules

The most typical rules of traditional dojos are to bow in and out of the dojo, never turn your back to sensei unless rearranging your gi, no talking when sensei is talking, be respectful to all students. Again, these rules are designed to create order and provide optimum training to all students. It is also designed to help with training the mind through mindfulness.

To train effectively in the dojo of your subconscious mind it is best to abide by these following rules of training:

Rule One: Become skilled in the use of your most powerful Mind-Sword: imagination.

There is an old Zen saying about how the same sword that takes life is the same sword that gives life. It is "*Satsujin no Ken*"(the sword that takes life) and "*Katsujin no Ken*" (the sword that gives life). You already possess such a life-taking and giving sword: Imagination.

Imagination is your longest Kiken, or Mind-Sword. It is your primary weapon in defeating old habits, creating new ones, and generating healing. Remember, from the preceding chapter that every thought or image you have affects every function of your body. Well, if you don't train yourself in properly handling Imagination, just like a razor-sharp Katana, you will hurt yourself or someone else.

Train yourself in its proper use and Imagination will give you life. It will give you healing and transformation. A key point to remember, however, is that Imagination is the total use of all your senses, not just visual. So, when using Imagination, it is best to engage all the senses.

Rule Two: Become skilled in two sword techniques (Nito-jutsu). Attach a strong emotion to your imagery. Miyamato Musashi, the famous Samurai, advocated the use of two swords over one because of its lethal nature. In Mind-Sword Hypnosis, you will do the same. When you attach strong emotion (your Wakazashi) to your imagery (your Katana) it makes it stronger and makes change and healing easier and faster. This is Nito-jutsu. This is the two-sword technique of Mind-Sword Hypnosis.

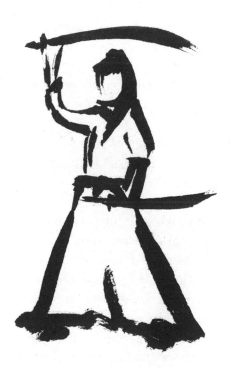

Nito-jutsu: Two Sword Techniques: Katana of Imagery and Wakazashi of Emotion

Since the subconscious mind is the home of your emotions, emotions tend to be a stronger and more potent source of energy than the conscious mind's reason or willpower. Physical force or determination, such as willpower, has less power to induce real change than emotional determination. So when you pair up your emotions with Imagination it makes what you imagine that much stronger...and makes healing occur faster.

Consider this. Have you ever tried physically forcing a two-year-old child to eat their vegetables? They clench their lips, turn their heads, stiffen their bodies, and swat at your hand. There is no way you are getting food into their mouth and odds are you are going to end up wearing the vegetables.

So, you can see, if you use sheer physical determination and try to force feed them until they eat, you may have some short-term affect, but still no real change will have actually occurred. However, what if you expressed joy and excitement and pleasure about eating veggies? You make a big deal on how delicious and exciting the veggies are. You smile, jump around and show sheer joy about how good eating veggies can be. Perhaps then, and only then, the child will sense this joy, making the probability of trying the veggies that much higher.

And when they do eat their veggies, reinforce it with more emotions of pride and how great it tastes. Shower the child with praise for being open-minded and you will have a child that will tend to try new foods and make parenting that much easier. This is what makes hypnosis effective. You spoon feed concepts to your "two-year-old" subconscious mind for it to sample. Once the subconscious mind has had the opportunity to sample the concept, it may find it likes the idea. If it does, it will act on that idea, reinforce it, compound it, and make it your reality. These concepts also apply to healing martial arts pain.

Rule Three: Have faith in the process...Don't try too hard. Faith is your tanto, the knife of your Mind-Swords. It is the smallest of your Mind-Swords and all you need is a little. Ancient Wisdom tells us that faith can move mountains. It can heal pain as well. You must have faith in the process. If you try too hard with the conscious mind (willpower) to make changes you will lessen the subconscious effect. In fact, overuse of willpower results in the activation of your subconscious mind's defenses. It angers the Fu Dog! More often than not this will produce the very opposite of what you want. This is also known as The Law of Reversed Effect.

Remember, the subconscious mind does not change easily, especially attempts at radical change. Things must be tested and proven before they are accepted. The will on the other hand, is temporary in nature, ruled by the ego, and wants everything now. The subconscious mind will automatically put up defenses to control the impulsive nature of the will. This prevents the will from causing damage by forcing untested changes.

The best example of this is trying to fall asleep when you have insomnia. You know the harder you try to go to sleep the less you actually sleep. So, what should you do? If you said, focus on something else, you are correct.

Also, you can't make corn grow by pulling on it. Just let the laws of nature take their course. Have some faith.

Rule Four: Practice daily (gyoji). To keep your Mind-Swords sharp and your skills at a high level, just like your martial art, daily practice or gyoji is essential. This is a key point. This is spoon-feeding that two-year-old subconscious mind a little bit everyday. I know I repeat myself, but it is important to remember that the Subconscious Mind responds to mental images, strong emotions, and faith. It is pure potential waiting to manifest. The mental image you form with your mind plants a seed of expected behavior. Eventually it grows into the wonderful garden of healing you desire.

In other words, if you expect to be sick, you will be sick. If you expect to be healed, you will be healed. We become what we expect to become. Each repetition or swing of your Mind-Swords regarding a suggestion creates less opposition to the next swing of the Mind-Swords regarding that suggestion. So, just a little bit of practice everyday builds great inner power.

As in the Chinese water torture, a drop of water is dropped onto the forehead of a strapped-down victim once a minute, but after the first few harmless drops of water, subsequent ones begin to feel like boulders smashing into your head or razors slicing deep. Just a little bit at a time and one drop contains vast power.

In other words, practice, practice, practice. Repetition is the key here.

Rule Five: Create rather than resist. Did you know your subconscious mind cannot see the negation or absence of something? For instance, right now, do *NOT* think of a blue monkey! An image of blue monkey crossed your mind, didn't it?

Think about this: "Not" is a word that has no image. Blue monkey is an image. As you recall, words are in the realm of the conscious mind and joined with ego and willpower. Images are stored in the subconscious. So, think about this: When pain flares up and you resist the image and feelings of pain by saying you wish you did *NOT* have it, the subconscious mind only "sees" you telling yourself to "Have Pain." It cannot see the word "NOT." And because the subconscious creates a physical reaction based on what it sees you will continue to have pain. In fact, you are sending direct messages prompting more pain. Ouch!

So, to prevent yourself from experiencing more pain, imagine comfort and healing instead. In your imagination, see and feel vigor and vitality. Your subconscious mind will then create physical and emotional reactions for comfort and healing. A hypnotic trick for this is to use what is called an imbedded suggestion. Here's how it goes.

Rather than say the word "pain," use the words "discomfort" or "uncomfortable" instead. Why? Remember blue monkeys? "Dis" and "Un" are not recognizable by the Subconscious, but "comfort" is. This is an example of an imbedded suggestion to produce comfort whenever you feel pain...excuse me, discomfort.

Rule Six: Act "As If." This is probably on of the most overlooked rules, yet one of the most important. To conquer pain you must begin to act as if you are already healed. As you recall, the subconscious mind does not know if what you imagine is real or imaginary. It perceives what you imagine as a real time event and acts accordingly. The more you imagine and emote that you are right now healed and full of vitality, the subconscious mind will begin to match those images and emotions with the necessary physical changes. Your emotional Mind-Sword must be one of "I am already healed" as opposed to "wanting to be healed." If you are in a "wanting" emotion this is what the subconscious mind will continue to produce…a wanting to be healed, never an actual healing. When you emote and image you are already healed and using your Mind-Swords in this manner you will manifest healing.

When I was healing my torn meniscus I would acknowledge my discomfort and say, "Hi, discomfort in my knee. I am feeling more comfortable today than yesterday and will feel more comfortable tomorrow. Today, I am at 85% comfort and tomorrow it will be 88%." Then on subsequent days, the percentages reached the 90's until it was at 100%. It really does work.

Go no sen, Sen no sen, and Sen sen no sen.

In Karate, and other forms of Traditional Japanese Budo, there are the concepts of "go no sen," "sen no sen," and "sen sen no sen." Go no sen is defending yourself after the attack as been launched. Sen no sen is intercepting the attack at the exact moment of attack, and Sen sen no sen is a pre-emptive strike. You strike as soon as you perceive your opponent's intent.

These strategies of self-defense are also relevant when you use your Mind-Swords You will receive training in these areas in the latter portion of the book. It is important simply to note that these strategies of Budo also relate to the use of your Mind-Swords and your ability to manage your discomfort.

I am sure you can relate to this. Some days your discomfort will feel as if it has launched a full-scale attack and hits you faster than a spinning backfist. The attack is here in all its glory and you have been taken down. This is when you will use your Mind-Swords in a go no sen fashion. Using my meniscus tear as an example, immediately after the injury I began to have lots of pain. It confused me and had me off-balance. Go no sen was then launched as the attack was here, now, and in-my-face.

On other days you feel discomfort arriving. You can sense its presence as it creeps in or begins to move quickly. Your awareness level of the attack is higher than in go no sen and so you simultaneously counter-attack with a sen no sen strategy. With my knee I could feel discomfort whenever I kneeled for meditation. The kneeling caused an attack of pain and I could then launch my own defense.

And lastly with sen sen no sen you may feel a bit of a twinge or an odd sensation and are now aware that if you don't do something quick you are going to be in tough situation. You launch your own pre-emptive strike. This is what I was doing when I acted "as if" my knee was already healed and getting better every day. I was taking the upper hand and using my Mind-Swords in a pro-active fashion, not allowing the discomfort to grow into a full-scale attack of pain.

*When your body separates into the four elements
upon death, where do you go?*

CHAPTER 8

Pure Raw Potential

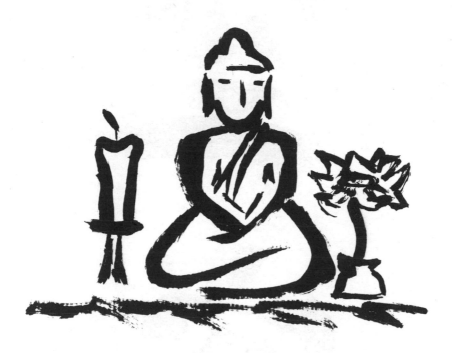

This is probably my favorite chapter in the book, because it is about Pure Raw Potential—it is about Emptiness, The Great Void, the Tao, the Mother of all things, the Supraconscious Mind. It is about manifestation and what makes the conscious mind, the critical factor, and the subconscious mind exist and function.

The Kamiza is the place of honor in the dojo and, in traditional dojo's, a Kamidana, or altar is present. The Kamidana symbolizes and pays respect to this source of pure, raw potential. The Kamidana can be simple or ornate in design and is considered another gate.

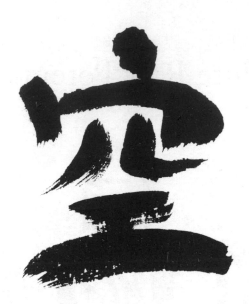

Kara of Karate

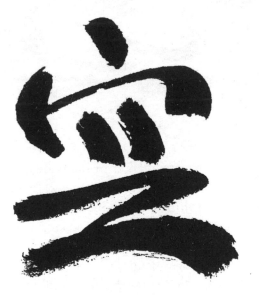

Ku of Emptiness

It is the dojo representative of the gateway to your Supraconscious Mind and core nature...and that is the Emptiness. This gate is unguarded and is passed through with simple faith, your third Mind-Sword.

Furnishings: The Supraconscious Mind, the Tao, or the Room of Emptiness is furnished with *Pure Raw Potential.* Its *purpose* or *function* is to create and heal. It is the source of all creation and at the root of the healing process. In fact, as an ego, you do not really heal. It is this supraconscious part of yourself that is continuously healing and creating. You just need to get out of the ego state (leave the genkan) and use your Mind-Swords properly. Then healing naturally occurs. Notice how a small paper cut on the hand heals quickly. You do not need to do much except keep it from dirt and not scratch the scab.

This Emptiness in Japanese is called *Ku* and is the same as the *Kara* of Karate.

You see, buried deep in the Japanese psyche is the Buddhist Heart Sutra that contains the famous saying of "Form is Emptiness, Emptiness is Form." It is chanted in Zen temples every morning. It pays respects to the creative supraconscious part of ourselves: Ku or Emptiness.

Emptiness here does not mean there is nothing here...it actually symbolizes and points to the creative source from which we spring and will return to upon this body's demise. Dojos, traditional ones that is, have a Kamidana to remind them of this fact and the sacredness of their martial art practice. I have mentioned this again, because it is needs emphasis. The subconscious mind cannot create without being an extension of Ku. *Emptiness is not no-thing but all things waiting to manifest.*

Karate, or Empty Hand, on one level means you have no weapons in your hand...your hand is the weapon...but if we apply the concept of Form is Emptiness, Emptiness is Form then what you get is the open hand as a symbol of Emptiness, the Great Void. It is pure raw potential taking the form of a fist, a spear hand, a claw, an eagle palm, a palm heel strike. It then becomes form but is still empty of any true form. It is a shape-shifter. It is pure raw potential just like you!

Rules

Believe it or not, the most basic rule for working with Emptiness, Ku, or the Tao is to "Please, Don't Feed the Bears." Yes, that's right. "Please, Don't Feed the Bears." In fact, for those of you who are looking for more reasons why Mind-Swords Hypnosis is unique, this is it. It is so important of a concept I have dedicated the next two chapters to its principles and practice.

Without speaking, without silence,
how can you express the truth?

CHAPTER 9

Please Don't Feed the Bears!

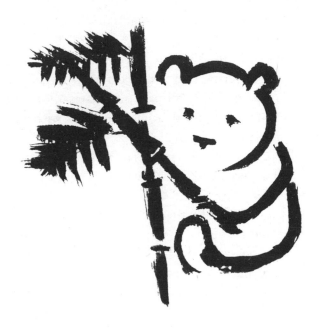

John, a seasoned martial artist and a very tough guy, came up to me while I was observing an Aikido session. We were at the 2007 North Central Wisconsin Instructor's Black Belt Federation's Annual Seminar in Rhinelander, Wisconsin. His right ring finger was heavily bandaged and he was holding his hand at shoulder height. John told me he had part of his ring finger amputated at the middle knuckle the day before. It was a work-related injury that did not heal well and so amputation became necessary.

He came over to thank me for teaching him about pain and how to work with it. He relayed the story how his pain meds wore off during the evening and he remembered, *"Please Don't Feed the Bears!"* Applying this strategy he was able to fall asleep without taking any more medications. If you have ever experienced an acute injury like this you know how it's throbbing can rob you of sleep.

Like John above, and David and Mary in the previous chapters, they experienced both pain and suffering. Pain is the physical trauma that aches, burns, throbs, or stings. Suffering is the anger, frustration, sleeplessness, sadness, or anxiety that comes along with feeling emotionally drained.

In this chapter, you will learn the conceptual nuts and bolts of how to work with your suffering that is concurrent with pain. When you stop and examine pain closely, all pain and its emotional turmoil are transitory. Once you learn how to adjust and work with pain it ceases to cause you suffering.

For the sake of learning the material in this chapter, I will refer to all emotional experiences that come from pain as suffering. The *"Please Don't Feed the Bears"* rule is the strategy you are going to use to take down your Bears of pain and suffering. To begin with, it is about realizing that suffering is nothing more than a huge grizzly bear and, when managed properly, will actually leave you alone. You see, it is possible to have pain but not to suffer.

As most people do, it is normal to equate pain with suffering since they are so intimately tied together. However, to conquer pain it is very important to see that pain and suffering are two separate entities. Pain is simply pain. It is the physical sensation of hurt. Suffering is your *resistance* to pain resulting in emotional hurt. The more you resist pain the more you will emotionally suffer and actually increase your physical pain. When you offer zero resistance to pain, suffering stops, and, in many cases, so will your physical pain. Yes, it does. So, let's talk about bears.

Remember as a child hearing the story of how to survive a grizzly bear attack? You were probably told when you encounter a grizzly bear there are two things not to do, right? One is to fight. Obviously you will lose, the bear will eat you and the bear gets fat. Two, is to run. Running provokes an attack. The bear chases you down, eats you and gets fat! So, you see, with your basic fight or flight instincts in the face of a grizzly bear (pain), you actually suffer (emotionally) more and make the grizzly fatter. Your pain increases along with your suffering and you get caught in a vicious cycle of pain causing you to struggle further. You then suffer, causing more struggling and increasing pain which causes you to increase your struggling leading you to more suffering, and so on.

Back to the insomnia example, did you ever notice the harder you try to go to sleep the more awake you become, and the more frustrated you feel? You are feeding the bear! The harder you fight or run to get to sleep the more frustrated and awake you get.

So what should you do? Stop struggling! Be still and play dead, no matter how much it hurts. This is the basic advice you receive to survive a grizzly bear attack. It is important to just let the bear be there, no matter how uncomfortable. When the bear is convinced you are dead, typically, the bear will cover you with mud or leaves and returns later. While he is gone this is your chance to escape and the bear did not get fed.

In terms of your pain, when you simply allow the pain to be present and do not fight or run, emotionally your suffering will decrease. You will be able to manage the pain more directly without all the clouds of suffering and your pain levels may actually decrease as well. As a martial artist you know it is easier defending against one opponent than two or three. Fighting pain and suffering together is actually trying to single-handedly survive a gang attack! When your suffering leaves and you begin to feel more relief and in control you know you survived! You won!

You are probably thinking right about now, "How do I play dead to pain…it hurts so damn much?" The answer lies in what the Samurai did… and what Budo, The Way of the Warrior, really means. You are now going to learn the base practice of Mind-Sword Hypnosis. All the hypnotic techniques you are going to do will be strengthened with this foundation. Like a good stance aids in a powerful punch, so will you need this stance. It is called Shikantaza.

Tozan shouted, "Don't just do something, sit!"

CHAPTER 10

Barebones Zen:
The Foundation of
Black Belt Hypnosis

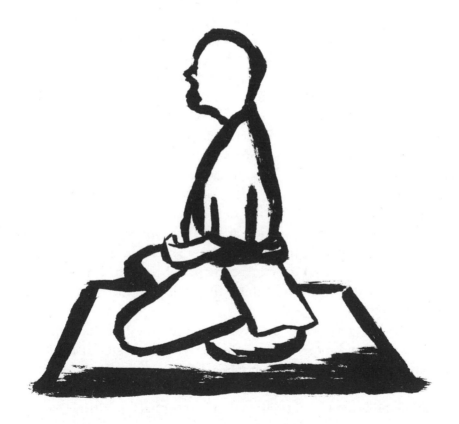

Just sit and watch what happens is a perfect way to describe Zazen.
It is The Way to play dead to the Bears of pain and suffering.

The shaolin monks practiced it and so did the samurai. They knew what they were doing. Zazen or Zen Meditation is the secret to just being here and remaining non-attached to what comes up, even pain. It is the perfect "play dead" exercise. In fact, Zen practice often talks about when you go to sit Zen you should have the attitude you have been laid in your coffin and the top is nailed shut. You are to just sit, without movement, and watch.

This is the practice of Shikantaza Zen. Shikantaza Zen is "just sitting zen." Shikan translates as "just this." Za is "sitting." So combined with Zen is "Just Sitting Zen." It is the simple practice of just sitting on a meditation cushion (or chair) while being mindful of your breath. It is also about paying attention to "what is" without struggling. As you learned earlier, "To Cease the Struggle" is the deeper sacred meaning of Budo. It is also part of the Zen Defense you will be learning about in the later portion of this book and the foundational stance of Mind-Sword Hypnosis.

Robert, a 45-year-old manager at a paper mill, was glad he learned how to cease his struggle. Robert was preparing to have his fourth back surgery and was in a heap of pain. He struggled and found it very difficult to sit or lie down for any length of time. He was also in jeopardy of losing his job.

He was instructed in how not to feed his Bears and in the practice of Zazen. He was very skeptical at first, but after six weeks of sitting and some simple imagery he wrote me a letter. He said, "When you first told me I needed to embrace my pain I thought you were nuts. But now I have found something that will help me the rest of my life. Thank You."

Over the course of six weeks his discomfort had become manageable and more importantly he was able to stay at his job. It is also interesting to note that when I followed up with Robert six months later he told me that he had stopped sitting Zen for a while and his suffering began to increase. He went back to sitting.

So, to get you ready, here are the basic instructions for Shikantaza Zen:

Sit in a comfortable upright position with your back fairly straight. Eyes half shut, tongue to roof of mouth. Place hands in lap and focus on your breathing in your lower tanden or hara (this is the area three inches below your navel and three inches in toward the back). Follow the inhalation and exhalation to the hara. When you lose focus, which is normal, simply return your focus back to the breath in your hara. Repeat for 30 minutes. When done, arise slowly and stretch. That's it! Let whatever Bears visit (thoughts, feeling, memories, pain) arise and be there. Watch them float away too.

This is like driving a car. Your focus is on the road (your breath) and while driving you watch scenery by the roadside (thoughts, pain, stress). Your "job" here is to simply return your focus back to the road when you realize you have been watching the scenery too long. You have to return your focus back to the road or you will go into the ditch!

Another way to look at this is by adapting Sky Mind. Or in other words, "Be the sky that watches." We all have this ability as humans to step back and observe ourselves. For those Karate-ka out there, Ku or Kara is also described as Sky Mind. The sky watches everything and is not bothered by what passes in front of it. Clouds arise and go away. Clouds can be thoughts, feelings, or pain perceptions. To practice Zen as the "Sky that Watches" is to practice the namesake of your art. It is the actualization of the Kara in Karate.

Zen practice is the core foundational practice of Mind-Sword Hypnosis. It will help you play dead to the Bears of pain and stress and enhance your hypnotic results. Zen Mindfulness practice changes your relationship with the Bear. It gives you the power to have pain in your life, but without the suffering. You see, as you stop resisting your suffering, it will decrease. You change the outcome and eventually gain a sense of empowerment.

"Playing Dead" is a skill, just like your Martial Art. Remember gyoji, or daily practice, is necessary to convince the Subconscious Dojo-Mind that this is who you are and what you can do. Gyoji is more than just daily practice; its deeper meaning is "essential activity." Gyoji is therefore practicing daily an essential activity, which in this case is Zazen.

But wait there is more. Remember that list you made way back in Chapter 1 about your pain? Pull that out. You are going to need it here. You are going to learn how to talk to your Bears. Yes, that is right, talk to your Bears. I know it sounds goofy, but talking to your Bears is a very important Zen Mindfulness practice. It is an essential activity you can do all day long and allows you to "play dead" in the midst of activity. This is a fantastic "street technique" that works extremely well.

When you feel stressed or angered or having pain, simply acknowledge the Bear and refocus on your activity. Here is what you say. "Hi Bear (stress, pain, or what you have listed) I see you. Come watch me _____(do the dishes, or my kata, or relax or answer e-mails)." Then focus on your activity and give it your fullest attention. When the Bear arises again, just repeat "Hi Bear...etc" and refocus. In this practice, your current "here and now" activity becomes the "road" you turn your focus towards. Eventually, you will be able to feel the Bears moving away and not be so bothersome. This is a wonderful mindfulness practice that is easy to remember and a powerful healing force. Practice for at least 21 to 30 days and you will begin to notice a difference in your life.

Zen Mindfulness is the learning to see how things are. Zen invites you to wake up to your life and its richness even if it is full of pain. It will help you positively transform your relationship with pain and stress. They will no longer erode the quality of your life, but enhance it. An important point to remember is that Zen Mindfulness is useless if you are trying to achieve anything with it. It is not a relaxation exercise as relaxation is goal-oriented. Zen practice is about non-striving and being open to what is happening now, without changing it, without resisting, without "feeding the Bears."

If you practice Zen with the purpose or goal of trying to get rid of pain, your practice will be impure, and I guarantee you will feed the Bears. Zen is about watching the unfolding of what already **is.** It cannot be done with a split mind. Pure Zen practice is to be aware and mindful of whatever you are doing with fully undivided attention! That is it. Whatever happens happens. You then take care of what happens next, until the next thing happens and so on.

Let's use the example of a football player. What happens when a wide receiver turns his head to look up field to the end zone just before the thrown football reaches his hands? He misses the ball and doesn't score, right? He now suffers (and so do the fans). His mind was divided between catching the ball and scoring a touchdown. The proper way is to keep the eyes on the ball, catch it, then run. Maybe a touchdown happens. How many times have you heard football coaches say, "Just take care of the ball"? This is very Zen.

If you practice Zen with one eye on your sitting and one looking for the Bears of pain to go away you will, in essence, "drop the ball." Pain and suffering will increase. So, have faith in the process of just being here. Let the Bears arise and let them move away as if they are clouds in the sky. Just watch and see what happens.

Part Two

Why is a mouse when it spins?

CHAPTER 11
Anatomy of Hypnosis

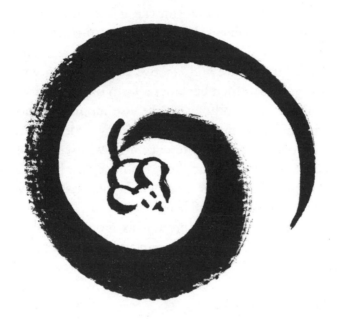

Tears of joy flowed down her cheeks. Jane simply could not believe her eyes. Ten minutes earlier her right hand trembled uncontrollably, and now, it was steady as a rock. The medicines didn't work. The physical therapies didn't work. In fact, her doctor's didn't know why her hand even shook. But now it was calm and under control. How did this "miracle" happen? What did she do? She hypnotized herself...with a little help from yours truly. Want to know how she did this?

Jane had learned the process of self-hypnosis. (In fact, all hypnosis is self-hypnosis as you learned in Chapter 1.) You must be willing to undergo hypnosis or it won't work at all, even with a trained hypnotherapist at your side. Jane had simply taken a walk through her Mind's Dojo, bowed in and picked up her Mind-Swords. I am going to share with you the Kobudo Kata or Self-hypnotic Mind-Sword technique she used to stop her right hand from tremors. After that you will learn the different components of the hypnotic process and how it is just like walking through the dojo to train

But first, you need to know you can indeed use self-hypnosis to solve virtually any problem. You can use it to simply relax and go to your "happy place" or expand your awareness and tap into your innate higher intelligence and creative ability. When you use it for this purpose hypnosis then becomes a form of meditation.

Self-hypnosis can also be used in those moments when you feel the need for the intervention of a higher power; it then can become a form of prayer. The subtle difference in these uses of self-hypnosis lies in HOW you direct your thoughts once you have altered your state of consciousness. All of these will be necessary for you to heal your pain and reduce your suffering.

So, back to Jane. She went through six movements or steps to be able to manage her tremors. They correlate with walking through the dojo. These steps are:

- •The Pre-Induction talk
- • The Induction
- • The Deepener
- • The Script or Patter
- • The Termination
- • The Debriefing

So, take a little walk with me.

The Pre-Induction talk is the listening and educational portion of hypnosis. This is the part you received by reading this book up to this point and will continue to receive up to the actual practice of hypnosis. Jane received pre-induction talk in my office.

The genkan is where you receive your Pre-induction talk. This engages your Conscious Mind and its logical and analytical powers, along with your willpower. This is your preparation to learning the rules of the dojo and how to conduct yourself with proper etiquette. It has been my experience that when you are educated about hypnosis and how it works, it will work better for you. Recall the old saying, "If you give a man a fish he eats for the day, but if you teach him how to fish he eats for a lifetime?" That is what the pre-induction talk does. It is teaching you how to fish.

This is also the time you give a numerical rating to your pain or what we call in the hypnosis biz, Subjective Unit of Distress or SUD. Typically this is a 0-10 scale, with ten being the most intense pain. For Jane it was at a 10. Just seeing her right hand shake so uncontrollably gave her the feelings of hopelessness and her high SUD rating.

The Induction is the beginning of the relaxation and mindfulness stage of hypnosis. It is where you take yourself into the hypnotic trance state and is symbolized by the bowing at the Gate of the Subconscious Mind. Here you are beginning to bypass the Fu Dog or guardian of the Gate.

Now, there are many forms of inductions. You will later learn Progressive Relaxation, which I consider a Power Technique and some quick-time inductions, your speed techniques. Jane was able to use a quick-time induction.

The Deepeners are conducted after the induction. This is stepping onto the formal dojo floor and proceeding over to the Kamidana to meditate. A deepener does exactly what it says. It deepens the trance with vivid imagery. It takes you to levels of relaxation you ever have rarely experienced. Jane used "The Staircase" Deepener which takes only about one minute to do. Jane had just entered the Subconscious Mind, bowed to the Kamidana and was ready to do battle.

The Patter is the script you use for healing. It is the meat of all hypnosis and comprised of both vivid imagery and strong emotion. Jane picked up her Wakazashi of Calmness and Security by recalling her "Happy Place." She attached these emotions to her other Mind-Sword of Imagery. It consisted of visualizing a heavy, yet cooling blue gel filling her right arm from the elbow to the fingertips. It was amazing to watch as her hand began to stop shaking and rested quietly on the arm of the couch. She was instructed to open her eyes and look at her hand. The tears began flowing. She had successfully used her Nito-jutsu, or Two Sword Technique. Her Mind-Swords gave her life!

Terminating the session is very important as well. This is where you are the most susceptible to post-hypnotic suggestion. This is where you bring yourself back to normal waking consciousness and return with changes imbedded in your Mind's Dojo. Jane's post-hypnotic suggestions included anchoring her experience with a finger squeeze of her middle finger and thumb of the left hand. Whenever she needed to calm her right hand all she had to do was squeeze her finger and thumb together. Then, presto, like magic, her right hand calmed down. Jane was returned to her genkan simply by coming back up the staircase. You will learn how to do this later in the book.

The Debriefing, like the Pre-Induction talk, is educational and analytical. You are back in the genkan. In terms of self-hypnosis, a debriefing is your analysis of the events or the scale of your pain so you can compare it to the Pre-Induction talk scale. Hopefully if you started at an 8 you are now at a 2 or zero. For Jane, she was a zero. Her hand was calm and she felt hopeful and elated. I got a big hug that day.

If you are helping someone else, it is also a time to listen to the person's experience and give homework assignments until the next session. For yourself, it is a time to develop positive affirmations to retain the healing progress you've made during the session.

Sensei asked the prospective student,
"Why do you wish to study?"

The student answered,
"To defend myself."

To which Sensei replied,
"Which self do you wish to defend?"

CHAPTER 12
Getting Ready

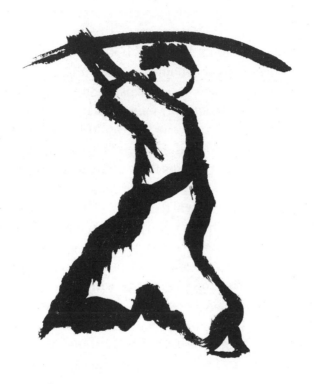

Hopefully, by now you have a general sense of the process for hypnosis. In the next few chapters you will be learning and doing more detailed work for yourself in each of the steps as you walk through your mind. In today's modern dojo, the changing rooms are considered part of the genkan. This is where you take off your street clothes, put on your gi, and prepare yourself for training. You make sure you have all of your protective equipment and you wrap your obi around your waist.

In terms of the hypnotic process, you have already prepared yourself by learning how your mind is a dojo and educating yourself about the myths and realities of hypnosis. As a hypnotherapist, this prep time is probably the most important part of the hypnotic process. It is here you create expectancy of change for yourself through a systematic process of reviewing your story of pain and reducing and eliminating your fears about hypnosis. It is important to learn, listen, and elicit your own imagery about pain and suffering.

I want you to do an exercise in preparation prior to entering the dojo. Write your story about your pain, how it has effected your life and provide imagery of how your life would be better if your pain was managed better or gone altogether. Get your internal pictures. In many instances, healing begins here as you become more intimate with your pain. As you write, there are a few positive statements I want you to jot down and listen/feel for any resistance. This will help you structure some of your story and keep you pumped for success. It may also provide some imagery and emotions you will need for the Mind-Sword work and strategies you will be doing later. So here are nine statements to write down and agree with or not. If you disagree or have some hesitation, go back and reread Part I of this book.

1) *It is my idea to use hypnosis.* It must be your own wish or desire. If a spouse, parent, or best friend is pushing you to do this, then it cannot be certain that your subconscious mind will be in agreement. Even if there is conscious compliance, the subconscious mind may be ready to sabotage the effort. The Fu Dogs will keep you out!

2) *I have a clear-cut goal for using hypnosis.* You must determine what you want to have happen. Make sure you aren't looking for magical answers or feel hypnosis contains super powers that can

help you rather than understanding that you are responsible for your own success. Simply make sure your goal is realistic and informed. Be aware of this.

3) *This is the perfect time for me to do hypnosis.* This is to determine your motivation for success. Are you having intense physical pain, sleeplessness or have an addiction out of control? Or are you just curious, seeking a thrill-ride because someone thought it was a good idea? Know your pure motivation. Although you may believe, be sincerely motivated, and have a ton of faith, is this the best time in your life to actually attempt it? Do you have extraneous distractions or stressors in your life that could sabotage healing? For instance, are you going through the breakup of a relationship or have just started a new job? These extra new stressors in your life may not lead to what we call keeping hypnosis ecologically correct. It must fit into the total picture of your life. Be clear on this and, as always, be honest with yourself.

4) *I am so motivated to change I would even pay for professional services.* This is a very important statement and an indicator of motivation. If you have some hesitation on this one, recheck your motivation. I have found people more successful with hypnosis when they have paid for the services than when I "gave" it away. People who are willing to pay are committed to change and less likely to be curiosity seekers. Odds are you are willing if you paid for this book. If someone has loaned you this book, check your motivation by asking yourself, "Would you pay someone to do this process for you?" If you only want to "try" hypnosis you will fail. It's like trying to tie your Obi. Only tying it will tie it. Trying is failure.

5) *I am very serious about changing my relationship to pain.* Rate yourself on a scale from 1- 10 how much you want to change.

It is also imperative to identify your level of motivation as it is directly related to your level of success. A level of 3 or lower will lead to failure. A level 5 will give you a 50/50 chance of success. If you can honestly report a 7 and up you are pumped for success. Be honest, though. The only person you will be fooling is yourself. Again, there is no try, there is only do.

6) *I wholeheartedly believe Mind-Sword Hypnosis will help me heal.* Once again ask yourself for a rating from 1 - 10. This correlates with the previous question. Faith is very important. It is your third Mind-Sword again. Be honest with yourself. Are you a 7 and up? If not, then you may want to reread the first parts of this book and build your belief systems first.

7) *I truly understand that with hypnosis my pace of healing is different than others.* One of the keys to success lies in individualizing every session to fit your world. Using generic "off the shelf" hypnosis scripts works for some people, but greater success comes with specific adjustments to your environment and lifestyle. The scripts you have been provided with should be tweaked and individualized to fit your specific situation. This triggers your personalized imagery more easily and results may come quicker.

8) *I have no fears doing hypnosis.* Check your gut and heart for this. If you have some fears, go back and reread the section about the myths and misconceptions about hypnosis. If you still have reservations then visit a professional or do some more research for yourself.

9) *I have honestly recorded my story of pain.* Make sure you write down your story. Writing it down is important so you have a reference for later as well as to draw out imagery and beliefs. I truly hope you wrote your story down. You need to remember what you have

done here, as you will need this information once you step on the Mind-Dojo's floor and pick up your Mind-Swords.

Since I am not with you in person, what you are going to do next is very simple. Obtain an audio cassette player or digital recorder and move onto the next chapter.

A monk asked Zen Master Yun-men,
"What is Buddha?"

Yun-men said, "Dried shitstick."

CHAPTER 13
Bow In

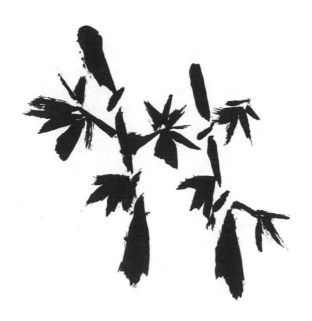

Now that your preparation is done you are ready to bow in and walk through the gate. This is the Induction portion of Mind-Sword Hypnosis. There are a variety of ways to bow in or do an induction. The most basic one, and the one I feel the most effective, especially for people who have never relaxed much, is progressive relaxation. Progressive relaxation is an exercise in mindfulness, which allows you to be aware of what you are experiencing with limited judgment. This is entering the area of "not feeding the Bears."

The other is like a speedy backfist, it is called a Rapid Induction. This is used when your pain is so uncomfortable sitting still for more than ten minutes proves extremely difficult. I will also use a Rapid

Induction on someone who is very nervous and to show him or her how easy it is to go into hypnosis.

Prior to any Induction make sure you are comfortable and won't be disturbed for 20 minutes. In order to induce hypnosis, and open the Mind's Gate allow yourself to sit comfortably in a reclining chair or couch, preferably a reclining chair. Lying on a couch tends to induce sleep rather than hypnosis. If your discomfort, however, makes it difficult for you to sit or lie down, you can do this standing as well. Many Qigong practices are done standing and are what I call a form of Chinese Hypnosis. I just want you to know that you have the freedom to choose what seems most comfortable for you when it comes to selecting where you will begin the process.

Some quick notes: If you are helping someone else and reading the scripts, your position is also very important. Sitting directly in front of the person to be hypnotized might feel too confrontational, sitting behind them might be too anxiety provoking, and lying next to each other might put both of you to sleep. The best location is to one side of the subject, but be certain they can hear from that side. I have had students whose hearing is only good with one ear.

The lighting should be soft, subdued, and indirect. However, if this causes undue anxiety, keep the lights on bright. Scented candles or incense can be nice and add a pleasant aroma to the room, but be aware that aromas can trigger powerful memories from the past. You can cover your eyes and ears but can't plug the nose in hypnosis, so be careful of the aromas in the room.

Gentle music is okay to play as well. Music made for massage, Reiki, or hypnosis works well, but keep it soft. No hard rock, punk rock, country music, or rap. The music must be in the background and not cause its own images as popular music tends to do.

Make sure you go to the bathroom prior to hypnotizing yourself. It is tough to get relaxed when your bladder is full and screaming at you to empty it. Also, if you are thirsty, get a drink.

If you wear glasses or contacts you might want to remove them. Some contacts can irritate the eyes and glasses begin to feel heavy on the face after awhile. Also give yourself permission to adjust your body during hypnosis at any time. You want to stay comfortable.

Progressive Relaxation

Now get out your audio digital recorder. In the paragraphs below is a script you can record for progressive relaxation. It is standard throughout the hypnosis world and can be modified to fit your particular temperament.

To get started, allow yourself to get in a comfortable position, either sitting in a chair or standing. Dictate the Progressive Relaxation Script into your recorder and then just listen. While recording make sure your tone of voice is normal, calm, and somewhat monotone. Certain words need to be made like they sound, for instance, as you say "down," use a down inflection. When you say "smooth" elongate the "smooooth." This is called squeezing meaning out of the words and helps you reeeelaaaax and the subconscious mind to respond to the emotional element.

Script for Progressive Relaxation:
Now while you are sitting here, please take a deep breath...exhale...let it all out...very good...now take another...very good...please close your eyes now...and allow yourself to relax...now it is totally okay if your mind wanders...and it is totally okay if you lose awareness altogether...the most important thing is your own relaxation...so just relax...feeling safe and secure...you are supported by the chair...and now taking in one more deep breath and exhale...become aware now of everything below your knees...relax your knees...relax your calves...relax your feet...relax the bottom of your feet...relax your toes...relax the tips of your toes...now feel again everything below your knees...allow them to relax...allow now this relaxation to gently flow into your thighs...relaxing your thighs... feeling them sink into the chair...now as you relax you may hear sounds coming from outside this room...these sounds will only help you relax even more...in fact every time I say the word "relax" you will find yourself

*ten times more relaxed than you just were...every time I say the word
"relax" you will find yourself ten times more relaxed than you just were...
now allow this relaxation to move into your hips...relax...relax now your
waist...allowing this gentle relaxation to move into your chest...and all
the organs in your body...allowing them to feel relaxed and peaceful...
allow your breathing to be more at ease and....relax...feeling more
peaceful...relax...allowing now this gentle relaxation to flow into your
shoulders...now down your arms...elbow...forearms...hands...fingers...
and fingertips...relax...feeling at ease...for this is your time...a time to feel
at ease...no-one wanting anything...no-one needing anything...feeling
this relaxation and comfort moving into your throat...back of the neck...
up to your scalp...moving over your face...like a wave of relaxation...
splashing down...feeling your eyes relax...the muscles around your eyes...
relax...relax your cheeks...relax your jaw...relax your jaw...feeling totally
wonderfully relaxed.*

You should be wonderfully relaxed at this point and ready for the
next step: The Deepener. You will learn this in the next chapter. After
becoming skilled in Progressive Relaxation, rapid inductions can be
used. Daily practice of rapid inductions will allow you to go deeper
and deeper into hypnosis faster and faster.

Rapid Induction….The Pretend Game

As I mentioned earlier, if your discomfort is very high and sitting
still is way too uncomfortable then try a quick or rapid induction.
The Pretend Game is one of my favorite rapid inductions and is very
effective. All you have to do is record the following script or commit
it to memory.

*Take a deep breath now, close your eyes and let out a sigh. One more
time, take a deep breath and sigh. One more time now, inhale, and sigh...
aaaahhh. And as you listen to my voice now, remember when you were a
little boy/girl you would play pretend...your toys would be alive, or you
were a superhero saving the world from evil, well, now I want you to play
pretend again. This time, I want you to pretend you are the greatest self-
hypnotic subject ever and capable of relaxing quickly, easily and deeply...*

And whatever I say to you now you will hear and understand and I want you to pretend that whatever I say to now will take immediate and quick effect upon your mind, body and entire spirit for deep and lasting change.

From here, you will simply move into "The Deepener." Yeah, it's that simple.

When the student is ready, the teacher appears.
But how do you know which is which?

CHAPTER 14
Mokuso

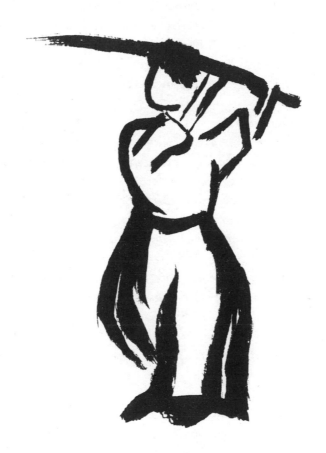

At this stage you are ready to step onto the floor of your Mind-Dojo. Deepeners are designed to assist you to settle your mind/body/spirit or Chi, if you will. Think of this portion as bowing in to the Kamidana and performing Mokuso, or a meditation. This will allow you to connect with the deeper Supraconscious Mind as well, which is, as you remember, the source of creation and creative healing abilities. Deepeners also engage the imagination and emotions more by preparing it for the actual hypnotic patter or script. The following Deepener is a classic. I use it almost 100% of the time. Why? Because it is so easy and effective.

This Deepener is called The Staircase. In this stage you imagine safely stepping down a beautiful staircase comprised of ten steps. With each step you take you will be guiding yourself down deeper into a state of relaxation and hypnotic suggestibility. Remember, this is to be recorded after you record the induction.

The Staircase Deepener:

...and now as you are so relaxed...lying there...allow yourself to use your imagination...imagine standing at the top of a beautiful staircase...a safe staircase you can walk comfortably down...there are ten steps...made of your favorite type of wood...your staircase can be carpeted or left bare... perhaps you have a guardrail...in a few moments time I am going to count from ten to one...and with each count see yourself taking a safe and easy step down, down, down the staircase...and with each step you will find yourself becoming more and more relaxed...you will find yourself becoming ten times more relaxed than you just were...so now... we begin...10...relax....9....feeling relaxed...8.....7..drifting deeper ...6....5....relax....4....3.....2....

1....at the bottom of the stairs...feeling more relaxed than you ever have before...

Another Deepener very similar to the Staircase is the Escalator.

...And now as you are so relaxed please use your imagination now... and see yourself standing at the top of a very safe moving escalator that is going down...down...down...to a more wonderful and deeper state of relaxation...and as I count from ten to one you will see yourself taking a safe and gentle ride down the escalator...so by the time I say the word one you will be at the bottom of the escalator...deeply relaxed...and so now see yourself step onto the escalator...10...9... you see yourself moving

down...down...down...8...7...6...deeper and deeper still...5...4...
down...down...down...3...2...1...feeling more relaxed now than you
ever have before...

And one more very simple Deepener.
And now as you are so relaxed and listening to the sound of my voice I
am going to allow you one minute of silence to drift deeper and deeper
into hypnosis...and so rest now, rest and relax until you hear my voice
again...(repeat one more time for a total of two times)

Using any of these three deepeners will help you drift and float
into a wonderful state of relaxation. Just allow yourself to let go. It is
time to draw your Mind-Swords.

Firewood never becomes ashes.
Firewood is firewood. Ashes are ashes.

CHAPTER 15

Kengeki: Sword Play

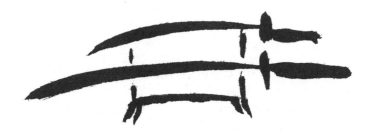

Now that your mind is in a highly suggestible state from the Induction and Deepener you have successfully stepped onto the floor of your Mind's Dojo. This is the fun part. It is time to "play Samurai" and draw your Mind-Swords. How you use your Mind-Swords is determined by the Scripts. This is the Hypnotic Patter. Listening to the patter in the scripts guides your Mind-Swords to the action it needs to take to relieve you of your discomfort. Just like dispelling you of a nasty nemesis. It is also likened to doing a Kobudo Kata. Just in case you forgot, visualization is the total engagement of your imagery (katana), using all the senses if need be, plus emotion, your short sword (wakazashi). This is Nito-jutsu, the two-sword method. Remember Musashi.

Go no sen, Sen no sen and Sen sen no sen.

As mentioned earlier in this book, in Karate and other forms of Traditional Japanese Budo there are the concepts of "go no sen," "sen no sen," and "sen sen no sen." Go no sen is defending yourself after the attack as been launched. Sen no sen is intercepting the attack at the exact moment of attack and sen sen no sen is a pre-emptive strike—you strike as soon as you perceive your opponent's intent.

In Mind-Sword Hypnosis, it is imperative to be aware of these moments so you can apply whatever strategy you desire. From the Catalog of Techniques it best for you to try as many of them as you can and see which ones tend to work for you when and how, as well as, was it during a time of go no sen, sen no sen, or sen sen no sen. This sensitivity and mindfulness, as you can imagine, will serve you well in the long run.

Mind-Sword Defenses

Swordplay involves certain defenses that coincide with the above-mentioned strategies. I have classified your defenses and scripts into three broad, and at times, overlapping categories. This, hopefully, will give you some structure, just like a Kobudo Kata. As you apply your Mind-Swords to slicing away discomfort and suffering you will be able to move them as if in actual battle. Now, don't get too caught up in whether you are following one category or another; just find the scripts that work for you. The three defenses are as follows:

1. Indirect Defense...think Aikido, Judo, or Aikijutsu
2. Direct Defense...think Karate's straight reverse punch...
3. Zen Defense...don't think

Indirect Defense is about not taking pain head-on but coming in at it from an angle. This approach utilizes identity change and change of focus. When you are in pain it is all consuming. It is all you can think about...trying to get rid of pain with your willpower, as you know, will not work. It will only increase the tension that comes from fight or flight and make pain worse. It is best to simply acknowledge the pain exists but then focus on your expected outcome.

For example, my daughter Hannah, age 24 at the time, severely sprained her right wrist. It felt tight, thick, as if she had a big wad of hard gum stuck inside it. The Indirect Defense is to acknowledge the wad of gum, but then to envision the end-state of a healthy wrist with free-flow of blood and chi...flexible and feeling 100%. The technique here is to not try and get rid of pain, but to envision what you want to create, not what you want to get rid of. Focusing on pain only increases pain...focusing on health will increase health. Remember Blue Monkeys!

Direct Defense is about straight-blasting the pain. Now this might sound like a contradiction to the Indirect Defense, but here you will focus on pain, and either directly numb it with an anesthetic script or "loosen the gum" with a solvent imagery so it flows away. This approach is best used AFTER you have had some success or practiced the Indirect Defense and getting some positive results, but it is okay to use it when necessary. As on the street, there are no rules. Just remember, if you are too early with this defense you do run the risk of exacerbating your pain rather than soothing it.

The Direct Defense I find works well for myself during Go no sen. I am already injured and hurting badly. I need a little relief so I can then apply some Indirect Defense and this makes flowing with the discomfort easier. I tend to think of this as my "pepper spray" for the Bears when they are too huge for me to handle.

The Zen Way is simply watching and letting the pain be. Whatever is is. This is truly playing dead to the Bears. Neither trying to run from it nor fight it. Just let whatever pain or emotions or thoughts about pain arise...and let them go by. Whatever pain comes up just let it rise. The Zen way takes time and practice, but over time is the best way to ensure long-lasting changes and true healing of mind-body-spirit.

Dainin Katagiri, my Zen teacher's teacher, used to say, "Zen practice makes your mind like teflon, nothing sticks." This includes pain. It will not stick. Without the Zen Defense your mind is like Velcro. Everything sticks.

I will always try this first, whether it is a go no sen. sen no sen, or sen sen no sen opportunity. It allows me to be more open and see more options as to how to swing my Mind-Swords if I need to do so.

Another Case Study

Mike, a blue belt karate student, suffered a punch to his lower left side and pulled muscles in the kidney region of his back. The hit was so hard, Mike stated, it literally took his breath away. He did not realize how badly he was injured until about an hour later after he got home. The pain was increasing and he wanted to vomit. He ended up going to the emergency room to get checked out.

Fortunately, he was only severely bruised with pulled and strained muscles, and not a bruised kidney. Needless to say this was very painful and traumatizing for Mike. For the first time in four years, he thought of quitting the martial arts. Here is the question for you: Was Mike in go no sen, sen no sen, or sen sen no sen moment? If you answered go no sen you are right. The attack is fully on and his Bears are increasing in size and numbers.

His pain was a hot burning across his lower left back. Unsheathing his Mind-Swords he used an Indirect Defense. Mike used the imagery of a zillion little people armed with fans cooling the burning sensation. He also envisioned a soothing blue over the area as the zillion little people fanned. This helped induce a cooling. He stated he could feel the difference especially after his session. Mike also listened to his self-hypnosis recording daily for one week and had remarkable success. He also used the Direct Defense of the Dit Da Jow script in your catalog of techniques. He envisioned the Jow directly going to his pain, numbing it and easing it...then eradicating it.

A few weeks later, after discussing his situation with me he instituted the Zen Defense, which included Zen meditation and mindfulness instruction. He was able to institute a regular Zazen and mindfulness practice along with his hypnosis. Mike began to feel more in control, even with his pain, and eventually became pain free in about three months. And he stayed in the martial arts!

Just as in actual swordplay, strategies do exist. The same goes for your Mind-Swords. You will learn in the following chapters how to use your Mind-Swords for an Indirect Defense, a Direct Defense and the Zen Defense to combat and heal chronic physical pain. There are many scripts you can use, but is important you know what type of strategy to apply to your discomfort. The following script is a classic for pain management and utilizes imagery of immersing yourself in a healing hot tub. It is classified as an Indirect Defense.

(To be recorded after the Induction and Deepener)

The Healing Hot Tub

As you are lying here...comfortable and relaxed...imagine for a moment... in front of you...a door...with a beautiful handle that turns easily as you open the door...this door leads to a room...a safe secure room...a Japanese bath...where there is a hot tub...it's been a long day...and your pain has accumulated...you can feel it throughout your body...perhaps in your neck and shoulders...or lower back...and then there's that one area that always seems to ache...take a deep breath...and begin to relax...see the hot tub...a whirlpool bath...with swirling warm waters...inviting you to relax...it is just outside of a resort lodge...nestled amongst the towering pines... with a breath-taking view of a nearby mountain range...crisp cool air... under the starry sky...private... serene...tranquil...inviting...steam rising quietly from the bubbling waters...the gentle chanting of monks in the distance...the soft popping of hundreds of bath bubbles...as the water boils and swirls in front of you...

*Take a nice deep breath...and now dip your feet...slowly into the water...feeling the warm soothing wetness...as your toes and ankles soak quietly...becoming warm, wet, and tingling...the heat soaking in... nicely...soothing and relaxing...you can notice if there is any tension, tightness, ache, pain, or discomfort...and...when you find it where it may be...you can feel the water's warmth soaking in...breaking up the tension...dissolving any tightness...massaging your aches...breathing in ...the warm waters...numbing the pain...soothing...swirling...warm waters...bubbly...steamy...relaxing... and your feet tingly, warm, numb, and wonderful...breathe...relax...dissolving pain...allowing it to move on...evaporating into the rising steam.

The process continues with your body being gradually immersed into the hot waters. Go back to the asterisk * and repeat the steps with the following body parts: lower legs and calves, knees, thighs, abdomen, waist and lower back, stomach, chest, upper back, hands and arms, shoulders and neck, jaw and facial muscles. It is also okay to modify this script to fit your unique needs as well. Remember this is an art form. All I am giving you is a springboard to work from.

Bodhidharma, the founder of the Zen school of Buddhism faced the wall. His successor, the Second Ancestor, stood in the snow, cut off his arm, and said, "Your disciple's mind has no peace as yet. I beg you, Master, please put it to rest."

Bodhidharma said,
"Bring me your mind, and I will put it to rest."

The Second Ancestor said,
"I have searched for my mind, but I cannot find it."

Bodhidharma said,
"I have completely put it to rest for you."

CHAPTER 16
Bow Out

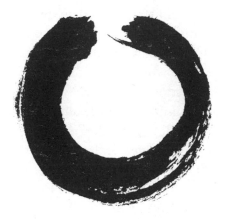

Ending the session involves bringing yourself back to normal waking consciousness. This is the time to acknowledge that your time in the dojo is done and you are, in effect, bowing out and preparing to leave. This is a very important part of the session as it is the time when your subconscious mind is most susceptible to post-hypnotic suggestion. Here's a script to help you get a good understanding of how it is done. Just remember to take your time.

Now that you are feeling so good...so relaxed...so comfortable...in a few moments time...I am going to count from one to ten...and as I count from one to ten...you will start coming back to waking consciousness...to this place and this time...and as you return you will remember all that was done here today...and carry with you the wonderful feelings of healing and comfort...remaining with you the rest of this day...into the evening...and through tomorrow...so now we begin to return...1...2...3...returning to this place...4....remembering now that whenever you feel discomfort...all you have to do in order to remember this place is squeeze your thumb and middle finger together... choosing any hand you desire...and comfort will return...5.....6...7...8 wiggling fingers and toes...9...and 10....you may open your eyes and move as you will.

I am often asked about how to use post-hypnotic suggestions. These are suggestions planted during the hypnotic patter and/or termination to help a client stay focused on their healing in a positive manner or to recall a healing "state." I tend to use them during the termination stage. I personally feel the subconscious mind picks up on it easier as you are "bowing out."

Post-hypnotic suggestions are typically tied to or anchored to a very strong emotion and imagery of healing and health. A majority of my clients respond well to kinesthetic anchors, such as squeezing a thumb and middle finger together. It is easy to do and to remember. You can add a combination of cues with this as well.

For instance, during the script of "The Healer," when the Healer is sending the client positive feelings of healing, simply tell yourself during this time that all you have to do to recall this healing is to squeeze your middle finger and thumb together of your left hand, take a deep breath and say, *"easy comfort"*...and you will be able to immediately recall the healing effect. Repeat at least two or three times to compound the effect. When you add a deep breath and saying "easy comfort," it helps give you a greater sense of control as well and has less chance of losing its effect when it is just a finger/thumb squeeze.

This post-hypnotic suggestion worked very well for Steve. Steve's back was killing him. He had had three surgeries on his lower back already and the pain was excruciating. In fact the pain was so bad, to get relief, he would lie on his bed with an electric heater spewing heat on his lower back. The burns on his back were horrible. He said the burns on his back helped distract from the pain in his discs. He also chewed painkiller like candy and would run out of his prescription before he could get a relief. This left him feeling trapped.

Using the finger squeeze technique as a post-hypnotic suggestion for relief and comfort, Steve was able to reduce his use of painkiller and the heater in as short as a two week period of time. He was very amazed at his success. The finger squeeze suggestion was that every time he squeezed his thumb and middle finger together it would trigger relief ten times more powerful than any painkiller, even morphine. It worked.

Another form of post-hypnotic suggestions is using colors. You can use the color "green" during the termination to help you remain determined in your goals of healing. You can use any color, but greens and blues tend to be more healing. Red might remind you of pain. (I use red for smoking cessation to remind people they now love clean fresh air in their lungs and would never put filthy smoke in their lungs. As you know, cigarettes have a lot of red in the packaging and the flame from a lighter and match are red.)

During the termination, the post-hypnotic suggestion can go like this... "1...2...3...*the color green will help you to remain calm and relaxed...4...5...*" and then move on to termination. You can suggest, like I just did, calm and relaxed, or you can suggest health and healing, or comfort and joy. Use your imagination. Just make sure it is framed positively. Bottom line, you simply anchor a color or physical motion to a heightened state of emotion so your subconscious will learn that this is what is right and good for you.

"When you stand up where does your lap go?"

CHAPTER 17
The Debriefing

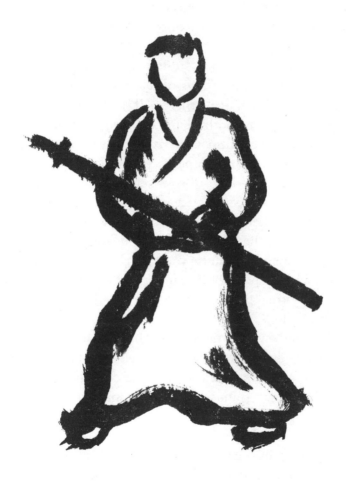

The Debriefing is simple. At this point you will feel, what one of my student's called, "gumbied," and not want to come back all the way to normal consciousness, but please do. You are now back in the genkan for some logical analysis. The Debriefing is designed for you to rescale your discomfort, or Subjective Unit of Distress, to show the power of your hypnotic abilities. It is also a time to write down any insights you may have gleaned or positive affirmations you might have thought of upon your return. When you have "returned" scale your Subjective Unit of Distress and compare it to your pre-session SUD. Celebrate your success with a loud, "Yes!" The word "Yes" drives quickly to the Subconscious Mind as it is emotionally charged. Try it.

If you are working with a student or friend, when they have "returned," validate their feelings of relaxation, loss of sense of time and sense of well being. Scale their SUD's as well. This is how they will know they were hypnotized and hypnosis worked.

The use of positive affirmations is also a very important part of your post-hypnotic plan. Properly phrased positive affirmations continue the "spoon feeding" of your subconscious mind. Think of it this way: You don't always practice your martial art in a dojo. Perhaps you are in your kitchen and carving a turkey when suddenly you feel like a Samurai with the sword and begin moving with your knife. Or as you walk through your house you find yourself suddenly throwing kicks or punches, especially if you pass by a mirror, checking your form. These informal practices keep your Mind-Swords sharp—so do positive affirmations.

For pain, a positive affirmation is "I am feeling better and better, every day. Every day, in every way I am feeling better and better." This is a classic one and I am sure you have heard it. One that I have used personally is, "Today I am feeling 80% comfortable and tomorrow I will be feeling 83% comfortable and more and more comfortable every day until I am 100%."

Other affirmations can be designed around your injury and imagery. For instance, if you suffer from fatigue due to fibromyalgia, the affirmation can be, "I am a person of infinite energy and health... and I am feeling great and feeling better everyday!" Or, if you are having a tight achy neck you can say, "I am feeling looser and more relaxed in my neck with each breath I take." Got it?

Now you will notice something about these affirmations I have used. Most of them are spoken in a positive present tense. Make your affirmations in the now tense, even if you are talking about feeling better tomorrow, couple it with feeling great right now. As I learned in college, a simple way to do this is to start off with the words, "I am feeling…." Keep your feelings or physical healings in the now… remembering to act "as if" all of this is now. And it really is.

Remember the Bears? A wonderful way to talk to them is using positive affirmations in this manner. "Hi, discomfort, come watch me use a positive affirmation."

And then begin your positive affirmation. Or, "Hi, frustration from lack of sleep, come watch me use a positive affirmation." It focuses the mind on what you do control and takes it off of what you do not control.

Part Three

Nanchuan saw two monks arguing over a cat.
Seizing the cat, he told them: "If any of you can
say a word of Zen, you will save the cat." Neither
monk could answer. Nanchuan cut the cat in two.
That evening Zhaozhou returned to the monastery,
and Nanchuan told him what happened. Zhaozhou
removed his sandals, placed them on his head, and
walked out. Nanchuan said, "If you had been there,
you would have saved the cat!"

CHAPTER 18
Mokuroku: Catalog of Techniques

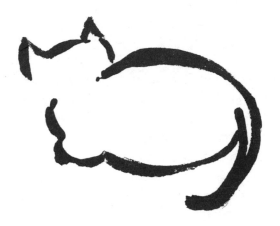

Many Martial traditions contain a written documentation of their techniques and can be called a catalog or manual. In traditional Japanese Budo it is sometimes referred to as the Mokuroku and presented as a teaching license.

Listed below are your Catalog of Techniques or Scripts. These are open to modification as you see fit, adjusting each script to your unique need. Earlier I had you write your story of pain. As you read through the catalog you will be able to see how to insert your unique imagery into the Script. In essence you are designing your own Kobudo Kata. It is like adjusting each self-defense technique to the situation.

The following scripts are the patter portion or swordplay. This is what changes. You can use the same induction, deepener, and terminator each time. It is the kiken-waza (Mind-Sword techniques) or script that changes. Self-hypnosis is like a kata. You open and close the same, but the kata itself is different. Scripts are the kata or as stated above, the Mind-Swordplay. Inducing the trance and deepening it are the opening bows and termination the ending bow.

Listing of Indirect Defenses

The Healing Dojo

Induction
Deepener
In a few moments time I am going to count to 3...and as I do so... see yourself projected back in time to the most famous healing dojo known...I will begin this count now...1 - 2 - 3. You are now standing outside the most famous healing dojo of all time.

(Pause one minute after each of the following suggestions)

Enter the dojo... and meet the warrior-healers who will be working with you...notice what they are wearing...how gentle they are...

You are now going through all of the diagnostic tests...these tests are gentle...no discomfort...

...Now the diagnosis has been completed...the warrior-healers begin the treatment...to help you dissolve your discomfort...to create healing... feel their powerful energy...their chi is strong with healing...and now you can see yourself being perfectly healed... participating with warrior-healers in the healing process.

See yourself perfectly healed now... leaving the ancient healing dojo... being projected back to the present time now... bringing with you the feelings and the energies which you have created.

Take a deep breath, open your eyes and stretch comfortably feeling the healing energy flow throughout your body

Terminate session

The Healing Katana

Induction
Deepener

...and now relaxing...continuing to drift and dream...allowing the subconscious part of your mind take more responsibility for your guiding your awareness...down...entering the gate of your mind...you find yourself now...in your mind's innermost dojo...it is spacious...feel the tatami under your feet...smell the incense from the altar...it is a place of healing...a place of awakening...and on the wall to your left...you see a katana...this is a special katana...it is your healing katana...a katana that can cut away discomfort...and create healing, comfort, and joy...it is truly the sword that gives life...

...and now seeing yourself taking the katana from its place...feeling its healing power surging through your hands...up your arms and permeating your entire mind, body, and spirit...you look now to the center of the dojo...and standing there is your discomfort...symbolized by a warrior... also armed with a katana...but a katana of discomfort and anger...

...facing this warrior...you assume your fighting stance...focused in a Zen-like calmness...your mind at peace...thankful for this opportunity to face your discomfort...seeing now your discomfort bring his katana overhead for a strike...you move to the side...entering into his attack... slipping by the edge of his katana's discomfort...and using your katana to cut him down...seeing him dissolve as you do so...and now...feeling a comforting feeling of joy and energy surge through your body...knowing you have control...you know you can face your discomfort and prevail... replacing it with comfort, peace, joy, and gratitude...you bow in respect to the discomfort...now returning the katana to its place...you prepare to return to this place...and this time...bringing with you the healing that has occurred...

Terminate session

The Healer

Induction
Deepener

...using your imagination now...I am wondering if you can see a large curtain hanging in front of you...and you may notice how easy it moves when you move it to look behind it...and as you look behind... just pretend for a moment you see a beautiful garden...flowers abound with the sun shining warmly...notice what it's like as you enter the garden...and feeling the cool grass under foot with each step you take... you walk and enjoy the smells of the flowers...the trees...the grass...in the distance, notice now what it is like as you hear a small waterfall...the water cascading over the rocks... and as you walk towards the water... glistening in the sun... you find yourself realizing this is a truly a special place...a healing place...where others like yourself have come...have come to receive special healings...special healings from ancient healers...that will come when you enter the garden...as you listen to the waters and see birds flying in the sky...notice now how you hear your name called...at first from a distance...then moving closer and closer...wondering who this is and now understanding ...it is your healer calling...calling you to come...as you see your healer...you feel comforted to be in the presence of such a wonderful person...you exchange greetings with your healer... making you feel safe...secure and hopeful...notice now as your healer places hands upon your head...you can see and feel healing lights swirling throughout your body...comforting any discomfort...healing wounds... making you healthier...seeing your body grow in strength, both inner and outer...your healer then moves hands to areas of your body that needs specialized assistance...feeling the healing warmth as healing energy flows into your discomfort...dissolving any traces of injury, illness, or long-standing discomfort...feeling thankful for your healing...you give thanks to your healer...feeling great gratitude for the work done today...

Terminate session

Direct Defense

Dit Da Jow

Induction
Deepener

....*relaxing now...drifting...knowing you are getting exactly what you came here for today...and that is to bring more comfort to your life... to help alleviate discomfort...and as you relax now...allowing your subconscious part of you to guide your awareness and healing abilities... imagine walking into a room...it can be arranged and decorated anyway you desire...this is a special room...a room of healing...just for you...so look around...what do you see...what do you smell....what do you hear... what is the floor made of...the color of the walls...what are they decorated with...is there music in the air...or the sounds of nature...and now as you explore your surroundings you notice a large bowl sitting on a simple table...as you walk over to this table and look into the bowl...you notice this bowl is filled with jow...the healing herb mixture used by martial artists all over the world...but this is a special jow...a jow made just for you...ten times more potent than any jow in the world...now be aware of your discomfort...be aware of its color...or perhaps texture or shape... or perhaps movement...so you now take some jow...either in your hands...or perhaps soaking a rag...and now placing the jow on any body part that has discomfort...gently rubbing the jow in...and allowing it's healing chi to sink in deep into your discomfort...turning into comfort...feeling the healing...feeling rough edges becoming smoother...or perhaps seeing colors of healing and comfort absorbing the discomfort...peace returning to the body's area...emotions calm...patience permeating your entire being... feeling alive and well...*

Termination session

Te-Katana Anesthesia

This is the technique I used to help calm the discomfort from my meniscus tear. I now use it often, especially when I have a headache or any discomfort for that matter. It gives great temporary relief, and in the situation with my knee's meniscus, permanent. Te-Katana means "Hand-Sword" and is a means to numb a part of your body that needs relief. Just like any technique, the more you practice the better you will get. Prior to entering into hypnosis for this technique, choose the hand that can reach the part of your body that aches. For instance, I used my right hand to be able to reach my left knee.

Induction
Deepener

Now as you are drifting deeper and deeper into hypnosis using the power of your imagination now...become aware of your chosen Te-Katana (the hand you are going to use to heal)...*and become aware now, just as your subconscious mind becomes aware of your remarkable ability to make this hand feel numb.*

See it now and feel it now becoming numb as if it has been injected with a powerful anesthesia...such as novocaine...feeling the hand becoming more numb...less aware of its presence now... and begin to notice its color, its weight, does it have a sound? Notice its remarkable numbness. In a moment I am going to count from five to one and with each count your hand is going to become ten times more numb than it was before. 5...4...3...2...1. Very good...now as you are listening to the sound of my voice and only to the sound of my voice feeling your hand becoming more and more numb...see yourself now taking your hand and placing it on the area of discomfort you are experiencing...and now, with your mind's intent, transfer the numbness of your Te-Katana to the area of discomfort...feel the numbness transferring...see the numbing action...if there is a sound hear the healing comfort moving into the area of discomfort...numbing...deeper and deeper...the healing agent of your

Te-Katana now takes effect…calming and soothing any discomfort… turning it into comfort and ease.

Feel this area now, numb and free of any discomfort…the numbing and healing agent of your Te-Katana now fully released into your (part of body) *feeling wonderfully released from discomfort and full of ease and comfort…and this comfort will remain with you as long as it is safe for you to feel this numbing action….and now as you prepare to terminate this section…this ability to numb your hand and any discomfort becomes increasingly easier and easier…so whenever you need to use your Te-Katana it will be available to you simply by thinking so…isn't that great?*

Terminate session.

Also, practice Te-Katana anywhere and anytime you need numbing action. The more you practice the better you will get. One more note: Pain is a messenger that something is wrong and so in cases of severe pain, numb yourself only for temporary relief and always seek medical attention. Numbing a serious injury when medical care is justified can do more harm than good.

Switches, Dials and Buttons

Induction
Deepener

Relaxing now, just relaxing your eyes and allowing yourself to drift… deeper and deeper…now allowing your body to settle down…I would like you to listen to my voice because there was once a young karate (or whatever art this person practices) student who was featured on TV documentary not long ago, who had learned to control all of his discomfort…He told the reporter that he learned how to go deep into his mind and slide open a special Japanese style door that led way down…down…a safe flight of steps...and at the bottom he entered a training hall...and along the front wall of the training hall...were many switches, dials and buttons...all clearly labeled...One for the right foot...one for each hand...a switch, dial and button for every part of the body...and he could see clearly the wires that carried the sensations from one place to another....all going through the switches...

...all he needed to do...was to use his mind's intention to reach up and turn off the switches, dials and buttons he wanted to...and then he could feel nothing at all...no sensation could get through...as he had turned off the appropriate connections...

And I am wondering now if you can see how he used his mind's ability differently from a martial artist who can simply make his body numb... he wasn't sure exactly how he did it...all he knew was...that as he relaxed and was non-attached like in Zazen...he could move his mind away from his body...moved outside it somehow...where he could be a witness...just pretending for a moment that you can watch and listen and drift...drift off somewhere else entirely...it doesn't really matter how you tell your subconscious mind what to do...or how you subconscious mind does it...

...the only thing of importance is that every time you want you know you can lose sensations as easily as closing your eyes, taking a deep breath and allowing yourself to drift...and as you are drifting down within... where something unknown happens tapping into raw pure potential that allows you to disconnect...that allows numbness and comfort to occur...and then allowing yourself to drift back towards the surface...and slowly now opening your eyes...as wakefulness returns...with comfort continuing.... and the feelings of safety and security remain and...the relaxation and ability to forget a leg, an elbow or anything at all, with no need to pay attention to things that are just fine, that someone else....can take care of for a while....there's no need to understand clearly how all this works as you drift in your mind...then return when it is time to enjoy the comfortable drifting upwards...where the eyes open and awareness returns completely...knowing you are in control...and you will continue with this practice, will you not?

Terminate session

List of Zen Defense

Just So

Induction
Deepener

*....Focus your attention by becoming aware of the part of the body that causes you discomfort (*name of body part*) Welcome the discomfort and... relax the muscles that surround the area, ...relax the muscles around the area, feeling them loose and relaxed...feel these muscles relax... and using your imagination... now see the area of discomfort (*insert description of pain*) ...and allow it to just be. Feel the discomfort and just let it be. Allow yourself to be curious about the discomfort...what does it feel like?... what does it look like?...does it have a texture?...a taste?...a color?... just be curious...like a monkey...examining a never seen before item... allow your mind...your focus to be open about your discomfort...being aware of your mind as you judge your discomfort...allowing the judging to be...feeling the emotions you have about your discomfort...perhaps it is anger...frustration...sadness...just let the emotions be here as well... welcome all that you feel...see...experience...now...with minimal judgment...no chasing away...no running away...just being present with your discomfort...feel the power you have now by just watching... being the witness of the discomfort...feeling in control...realizing you are not your discomfort...it is just something here...like a cloud...or a tree...not you...but just here...no need to do anything with it...it will move on its own...allow the discomfort to do its job of healing...and you just watch...just watch...now just stay the witness...trusting your body's wisdom to heal...and rest in the comfort of being here now...open and free...*

Breaking the Trance of False Self: Ku

Induction
Deepener

...as you are relaxing so nicely now...drifting deeper and deeper...become aware now of your intention for this meditation...to be aware and awake to benefit all beings...seen and unseen.

...with the alertness of a ninja spy...or the clear insight of a Zen master...slowly become aware of the person you call "I"...who is this "I" who is listening...who is this "I" who is thinking now....who is feeling now...who is this "I"....allowing that subconscious part of you now to take over...as you get used to drifting deeper and deeper...wondering now

how does this "I" come into existence....how does it appear to you....is your "I" a creation of your own mind...or is it something independent.... floating...drifting...

again wondering now if can you locate the "I" you call you...in your body...beginning now to examine your body...is this "I" in your head?... your scalp?...your eyes?...your heart?...stomach?...shoulders?... back?... legs?....feet?...can you find the "I" in your body?...is it in your cells?...is it in your atoms?...or is it the energy that moves your body...sooner or later you now are aware of your breathing wondering ...is your "I" here?... does it still feel very strong?...is it easy to feel now?...or more ...

how about your thoughts now...is your "I" here...as you continue your journey of floating and drifting with your feelings....what about them.... is your "I" in your feelings of love...is it in your thoughts of anger...is it in excitement....is it in calmness...is it in practicing your favorite self-defense skill...how about your dreams...is the "I" here...

and now when you take a few moments .... a few moments of silence... exploring other places to look for the "I" you call yourself...wondering where is it....what does it look like....feel like...is it solid...or transparent...is it in your body...or outside of your body...so remember now take a moment of silence and explore trusting your mind's ability to float and sink deeper and deeper into exploration...until you hear my voice again...

(let one minute pass)

Now, you are doing a fine job...relaxing in this special way...I want you now to become aware again of your body now...from the top of your head to the tips of your toes...pretending now that your body is disintegrating... all of the atoms separating and floating apart and away...seeing all the billions of subatomic particles scattering throughout the universe...see this happening to you now...and now do the same with your thoughts, feelings, sensation...see them disintegrate, separate and float into space... separating...floating away... into space...

stay with this experience...and when your thoughts wander...please return them to this experience...if feelings or other sense perceptions arise... be aware of them...where do they exist in your body?...where do they exist in your mind?...how does it exist?...how can it exist?...

now you know you do exist...allow yourself to experience...this emptiness...this pure raw potential...which is in fact an interconnectedness with all phenomenon...your true nature...is this emptiness...not dependent upon mind or body...but interconnected to them....

again...allow your self some time of silence...exist in this state....

(allow one minute)

allow yourself now to reconnect with your mind, thoughts, feelings.... feeling them more solid now...your body as well....reintegrating them back into the existence you know...and as you become more and more aware of your mind, body, thoughts, and feelings...you are feeling better and better...calm and comforted...refreshed and renewed...

...so now continue feeling energized...for in a few moments time.... this session will conclude....bringing you back to this place and this time....feeling refreshed...calm...at peace with yourself....knowing a great healing has occurred...and will continue to occur....

Termination session

Fukanzazengi: Universal Instructions for Zazen

by Dogen Zenji, Founder of Soto Zen in Japan.
(Translation by Rev. Nonin Chowaney)

This Sutra is recited in Soto Zen temples across the world, typically after the last meditation period of the day. It is more than just instructions on how to sit Zen. Fukanzazengi points you directly to that place where you are free from all suffering and distress. Listening to this sutra and practicing its words is a wonderful way to manage your discomfort as well as your life. It is a powerful hypnotic script.

Induction
Deepener

The Way is basically perfect and all pervading. How could it be contingent upon practice and realization? The Dharma-vehicle is free and untrammeled. What need is there for concentrated effort? Indeed, the whole body is far beyond the world's dust. Who could believe in a means to brush it clean? It is never apart from one, right where one is. What is the use of going off here and there to practice? And yet, if there is the slightest discrepancy, the Way is as distant as heaven from earth. If the least like or dislike arises, the Mind is lost in confusion. Suppose one gains pride of understanding and inflates one's own enlightenment, glimpsing the wisdom that runs through all things, attaining the Way and clarifying the Mind, raising an aspiration to escalade the very sky. One is making the initial, partial excursions about the frontiers but is still somewhat deficient in the vital Way of total emancipation.

Need I mention the Buddha, who was possessed of inborn knowledge? The influence of his six years of upright sitting is noticeable still. Or Bodhidharma's transmission of the mind-seal?—the fame of his nine years of wall-sitting is celebrated to this day. Since this was the case with the saints of old, how can we today dispense with negotiation of the Way?

You should therefore cease from practice based on intellectual understanding, pursuing words, and following after speech, and learn the backward step that turns your light inwardly to illuminate your self. Body and mind of themselves will drop away, and your original face will be manifest. If you want to attain suchness, you should practice suchness without delay.

For sanzen, a quiet room is suitable. Eat and drink moderately. Cast aside all involvements and cease all affairs. Do not think good or bad. Do not administer pros and cons. Cease all the movements of the conscious mind, the gauging of all thoughts and views. Have no designs on becoming a Buddha. Sanzen has nothing whatever to do with sitting or lying down.

At the site of your regular sitting, spread out thick matting and place a cushion above it. Sit either in the full-lotus or half-lotus position. In the full-lotus position, you first place your right foot on your left thigh and your left foot on your right thigh. In the half-lotus, you simply press your left foot against your right thigh. You should have your robes and belt loosely bound and arranged in order. Then place your right hand on your left leg and your left palm (facing upwards) on your right palm, thumb-tips touching. Thus sit upright in correct bodily posture, neither inclining to the left nor to the right, neither leaning forward nor backward. Be sure your ears are on a plane with your shoulders and your nose in line with your navel. Place your tongue against the front roof of your mouth, with teeth and lips both shut. Your eyes should always remain open, and you should breathe gently through your nose.

Once you have adjusted your posture, take a deep breath, inhale and exhale, rock your body right and left and settle into a steady, immobile sitting position. Think of non-thinking. How do you think of not-thinking? Non-thinking. This in itself is the essential art of Zazen.

The Zazen I speak of is not learning meditation. It is simply the Dharma gate of repose and bliss, the practice-realization of totally culminated enlightenment. It is the manifestation of ultimate reality. Traps and snares can never reach it. Once its heart is grasped, you are like the dragon when he gains the water, like the tiger when she enters the mountain. For you must know that just there (in Zazen) the right Dharma is manifesting itself and that, from the first, dullness and distraction are struck aside.

When you arise from sitting, move slowly and quietly, calmly and deliberately. Do not rise suddenly or abruptly. In surveying the past, we find that transcendence of both unenlightenment and enlightenment, and dying while either sitting or standing, have all depended entirely on the strength (of zazen).

In addition, the bringing about of enlightenment by the opportunity provided by a finger, a banner, a needle, or a mallet, and the effecting of realization with the aid of a hossu, a fist, a staff, or a shout, cannot be fully understood by discriminative thinking. Indeed, it cannot be fully known by the practicing or realizing of supernatural powers, either. It must be deportment beyond hearing and seeing—is it not a principle that is prior to knowledge and perceptions?

This being the case, intelligence or lack of it does not matter: between the dull and the sharp-witted there is no distinction. If you concentrate your effort single-mindedly, that in itself is negotiating the Way. Practice-realization is naturally undefiled. Going forward (in practice) is a matter of everydayness.

In general, this world, and other worlds as well, both in India and China, equally hold the Buddha-seal, and over all prevails the character of this school, which is simply devotion to sitting, total engagement in immobile sitting. Although it is said that there are as many minds as there are persons, still they all negotiate the way solely in Zazen. Why leave behind the seat that exists in your home and go aimlessly off to the dusty realms of other lands? If you make one misstep, you go astray from the Way directly before you.

You have gained the pivotal opportunity of human form. Do not use your time in vain. You are maintaining the essential working of the Buddha-Way. Who would take wasteful delight in the spark from the flint stone? Besides, form and substance are like the dew on the grass, destiny like the dart of lightning—emptied in an instant, vanished in a flash.

Please, honored followers of Zen, long accustomed to groping for the elephant, do not be suspicious of the true dragon. Devote your energies to a way that directly indicates the absolute. Revere the person of complete attainment who is beyond all human agency. Gain accord with the enlightenment of the Buddhas; succeed to the legitimate lineage of the ancestors' Samadhi. Constantly perform in such a manner and you are assured of being a person such as they. Your treasure-store will open of itself, and you will use it at will.

Terminate session

Cease the Struggle

Induction
Deepener

Name, *you might find yourself beginning to understand fully just how easily you can cease the struggle with discomfort. As a warrior, a person can easily imagine the many possibilities of defending yourself from the onslaught of discomfort… and as you allow your mind now to drift and float relaxing into comfort which means you are gaining health and vitality…as soon as you discover the ease with which you can cease the struggle with discomfort and turn to comfort in your daily life, you will find yourself smiling more and returning to your training with full vigor and comfort and joy…knowing you have control as a warrior who has put away his swords and can rest in relief, comfort, and ease. So now just pretend for a moment that you're the kind of warrior who can master the skills of visualization and there's no need to understand clearly how all of this works, which means all you have to do is practice visualizing in this special way allowing comfort to take over your mind and body and you will soon discover how easy it is to cease the struggle and move into relief and vigor. What would it be like if you found yourself feeling totally free of any discomfort and walking the way of the warrior naturally and easily? When you listen to these words will you soon realize how natural comfort is your natural way of being and becoming…and when you are listening to these words allowing yourself to continue to drift and float deeper and deeper into comfort…feeling joy returning to your spirit you could just pretend, if even for a moment of being in total health, totally healed and full of comfort, couldn't you? As you get used to relaxing and ceasing the struggle with your discomfort your wisdom warrior spirit takes over more and more and you will find it extremely easy to heal and be of good health…all discomfort dissolving and drifting away…like a dream after you awake….just dissolving and drifting away…and you are left with calmness and comfort. You should remember now that comfort is a natural state of being and just allow it to happen and enjoy the process of healing and so now each and every time you practice this new skill of visualizing comfort your level of skills and comfort will continue to grow…there is no need to struggle anymore as this is a thing of the past… your path is now clear and easy allowing comfort and healing to being your most natural state of mind, body, and spirit…and now you will continue in this manner, won't you?*

Terminate session

Discomfort Drifts Away

Induction
Deepener

You should remember now as you become less aware of your physical body…and you become more aware of your own innate subconscious mind that really knows everything about your health and healing abilities… and the subconscious part now opens like a lotus to the sky…receiving and accepting and above all acting upon all the positive images and emotions that I suggest for you now…and as you listen to my voice you drift deeper and deeper now…your subconscious mind becoming more and more alert…it is as if your attention is being focused on healing discomfort now which makes it easier to heal now…repairing and regenerating any part of your body that is uncomfortable…allowing you to see life now in a positive manner which is for your highest good and ease and comfort…

Noticing now as you drift deeper and deeper into a peaceful calm... as your body rests into comfort...and imagining now yourself in a most beautiful place...noticing what it's like when you feel safe and secure here...calm and comfortable here...your mind and body at rest...and it's a good thing to be aware that you can return here at any time you desire... and I know you're wondering if you can find those feelings of comfort so you can drift deeper and deeper now...

You may notice now as you drift and float deeper into this place... the soft ground beneath your feet as you walk...the wind gently flowing through the trees...the sunlight warming your skin...and there's no need to understand clearly how you can easily let go and rest ever so deeply now...until...

Finding yourself now beside a crystal clear pool of healing waters... where you find yourself dipping a hand into the water feeling its heated and healing nature...steam rising effortlessly from the surface...bubbles coming forth now from the depths of this safe and serene pool...you may be wondering what it would feel like to dip your entire body into this warm and comfortable blanket of healing moisture...

And so now...you now find a gentle rocky ledge from which to gently lower your body into the waters of the pool...and when you find yourself up to your chest...you are feeling safe and secure...able to float effortlessly with the bubbles of the pool...feeling the bubbles now caressing your body...massaging it...comforting it...wondering now what it would feel like having the heated waters relaxing you deeper and deeper...bringing you calm and comfort...your body feeling at ease...relaxed...loose...being gently massaged and kneaded by the gentles waves of the pool...penetrating deeply into those areas needing comfort...deep into the muscles...deep into the joints...deep into the bones themselves...calming you...relaxing you... healing you...all discomfort being washed away by the healing forces of the water...peace and comfort permeate throughout...

As soon as you settle in even deeper now as the waters continue their massage...calming and comforting you...every part of your body from the top of your head to the tips of your toes is now free from all discomfort... feeling now more peaceful...which means you are healing deeply now...

and repairing and healing all discomfort...I am going to give you a moment or two of silence to rest ever more deeply into the pool...and when I speak to you again in a few moment time you will find yourself so relaxed...so comforted...so free...all discomfort floated away...

(give yourself about one to two minutes of silence)

...and now each and every time you practice this type of relaxation you will find your ability to drift and float and enjoy the comfort of the waters increase tenfold...so continue relaxing now...feeling warm and comfortable...

Terminate session

The Three Battles (1): Suffering, Sleeplessness and Sadness

Induction
Deepener

Now tell yourself that every word I say now is going to fix itself in your inner mind, body, and spirit...and be sealed, stamped, engraved, and programmed into it, so that it will stay there, sealed, stamped, engraved and programmed...and that without your will or knowledge, accepting no laziness from the deep part of you, will obey with your mind, body and spirit. And all these words will be for your benefit and your benefit only.

From this point forward, physically as well as mentally and spiritually, you are now enjoying excellent health more than you have ever been able to experience. You are a healthy and rapidly healing being with remarkable gifts of recovery from injury, illness and discomfort. In fact, you find it extremely easy to heal, finding your mind, body and spirit enjoying wonderful comfort from the time you awake till you fall asleep in the evening. (repeat two more times)

Furthermore, from now on and every night whenever you wish to go to sleep you will sleep deeply, contently, and restfully with total comfort of body, mind, and spirit. Your dreams will be full of healing wisdom and comfort and upon waking you will feel wonderfully refreshed, cheerful, and optimistic in every way. (Repeat two more times)

And even better now, as you go through your day, your mood will be one of continuing and renewed optimism full of life and vigor. You look forward to the day ahead and completing your duties with good cheer and a smile that comes deep from within…and all of these suggestions will be easy for you to do. (Repeat 2 more times)

And from this point forward, you will find daily visualizing in this special way easy and stay positive with your thoughts, repeating to yourself at least 21 times, 21 times per day, "I am a warrior who is happy, healthy, and well-rested." (Repeat this "I am…" at least 21 times or more during the script)

And so, from this point forward your deep inner mind, body and spirit has accepted these suggestions for your better good.

Terminate session

The Three Battles (#2- Extended Version)

If you saw Bruce Lee's *Game of Death* and his epic battle against an array of foes to reach the top of the pagoda where Kareem Abdul-Jabbar was awaiting…go see it. This script is based on the model. Here you will use three levels each representing either sleeplessness, sadness, or suffering. The gender is male based…please feel free to insert female if you are female.

Induction
Deepener

As you relaxing now I want you to know you are getting out of this relaxation exactly what you came here for today. For you want to feel happier, sleep better, and be more comfortable in your body, mind, and spirit. And these wonderful things are happening to you now as you listen to my voice…

So now I want you to see a tall three story pagoda temple…don't worry if you can't see the temple clearly, just allow time to pass…and as you see the temple you can see a man standing at the bottom of the temple…

The man at the bottom of the temple is looking very sad and unhappy. He is sad and unhappy because he is in pain…at least five times more than you are yourself. He can't sleep at night because of the pain, he is restless and fatigued throughout the day and just wants his life back. He is a very sad and miserable man because of his pain.

Now realize just as the sad man realizes that the temple is a symbol of his three battles he faces of sleeplessness, sadness, and suffering. It is a symbol of his struggles to feel healthy and well rested. Each floor represents one of the three battles. The bottom floor contains the defender of sleep, the second of suffering and the third of sadness.

And now notice again, just as the sad man notices, he sees another man standing on the top floor of the pagoda temple. This man is healthy, practicing his martial art. He is in total comfort and well rested from having a wonderful night's sleep. He is happy and content because he conquered the defenders of each floor of the pagoda's three floors. He battled his way to the top and won! Notice how happy, healthy, and content he is.

Now notice the man at the bottom of the pagoda. Notice how sad and unhappy he is. (pause)

Now, notice the man at the top of the pagoda. Notice how happy and healthy he is.

Now once again, notice the sad man at the bottom of the temple and notice now how determined he is to do battle. He has decided to battle each of the three defenders. He gathers his weapons and enters the bottom floor. Now see him defeating sleeplessness and feeling refreshed and now he moves to the next floor.

See him now defeating suffering and feeling more comfort now, feeling victorious, moving to the third floor and now see him defeating sadness, feeling happy and content. See him now standing next to the other happy man at the top of the pagoda temple. See how similar they both look, happy, comfortable, and well rested. Notice now how both are so similar

they look like identical twins. Now merge the two men into one figure...
...and see that this man is now you... feel the health, optimism, and
rest. Feel the exhilaration of conquering your sleeplessness, suffering, and
sadness...you deserve to be here and to help keep you at the top of the
pagoda this is what is happening to you....

Firstly, now tell yourself that every word I say now is going to fix itself
in your inner mind, body, and spirit...and be sealed, stamped, engraved,
and programmed into it, so that it will stay there, sealed, stamped,
engraved and programmed...and that without your will or knowledge,
accepting no laziness from the deep part of you, will obey with your mind,
body, and spirit. And all these words will be for your benefit and your
benefit only.

From this point forward, physically as well as mentally and spiritually,
you are now enjoying excellent health more than you have ever been able to
experience. You are a healthy and rapidly healing being with remarkable
gifts of recovery from injury, illness, and discomfort. In fact, you find
it extremely easy to heal, finding your mind, body, and spirit enjoying
wonderful comfort from the time you awake till you fall asleep in the
evening. (Repeat 2 more times)

Furthermore, from now on, and every night whenever you wish to go
to sleep, you will sleep deeply, contently, and restfully with total comfort
of body, mind, and spirit. Your dreams will be full of healing wisdom and
comfort and upon waking you will feel wonderfully refreshed, cheerful,
and optimistic in every way. (Repeat 2 more times)

And even better now, as you go through your day, your mood will be
one of continuing and renewed optimism full of life and vigor. You look
forward to the day ahead and completing your duties with good cheer and
a smile that comes deep from within...and all of these suggestions will be
easy for you to do. (Repeat 2 more times)

And from this point forward you will find daily visualizing in this
special way easy and stay positive with your thoughts, repeating to yourself
at least 21 times, 21 times per day, "I am a warrior who is happy, healthy,
and well rested." (Repeat this "I am.." at least 21 times or more during
the script)

And so, from this point forward your deep inner mind, body and spirit has accepted these suggestions for your better good. And you are better for it…are you not?

Terminate session

Turning Discomfort to Comfort to Joy

Induction
Deepener

You might realize your discomfort turning into comfort turning into joy after you spend some time relaxing in this special way…and as you allow yourself to relax with your thoughts and begin to notice how calm and comfortable your body is already beginning to feel you'll be able to have more comfort in your life…as soon as you discover the ease with which you can turn discomfort into comfort you'll feel amazed about the fact you put in hardly any effort at all…

What would it be like if you found yourself being able to have tremendous joy in your life simply by relaxing and visualizing in this way, absorbing what you learn here naturally which means you are well on the way to healing your discomfort. Comfort returns, but you don't have to use this visualizing right away as long as you simply allow your mind and body to relax and extend your intentions to comfort and joy.

When you hear my voice you will soon realize as well how natural and easy it is for your body to heal once relaxation is evident in your life… and it is now because you are listening to these words of comfort, turning discomfort to comfort to joy…and it is easy…which means that your healing takes place on a higher plane of existence than you ever thought of before…If you were to understand how easy healing is how much more would you do this exercises of visualizing and relaxing?

Have you ever started to learn something new and discovered how easy and joyful it can be? Just pretend for a moment now that you're the kind of person that can master inner healing and easily turn discomfort into comfort into joy. What would that be like? Yes, what would it feel like? How does it look? Who is with you? What are you doing now that you are full of joy?

When you find yourself now full of comfort and joy will you now be really inspired to continue practicing these exercises? Of course you will. Imagine—just imagine what it would be like to have this type of power and how your martial skills will also improve. Discomfort will no longer be an issue for you as you now have the skills and abilities to change discomfort to comfort to joy…and so, now each and every time you practice this form of relaxation your skill levels increase and you enjoy doing it even more. You should remember this is a natural thing do as well as easy.

Terminate session

All that you need is here...now.
Where else can you look?

CHAPTER 19
Weight Loss

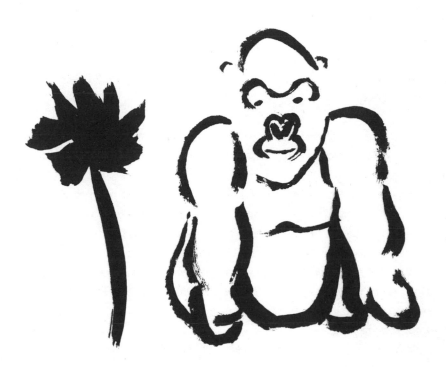

As most of us know, excessive weight can bring excessive pain to injuries, especially if they are joint-related. Knees, hips, and ankles hurt more, as well as the back. For martial artists who typically are in good shape you might find yourself gaining weight if you can't practice as often as you used to and you slip into a depressed state of mind whereby you emotionally eat to cover up the suffering.

The key is not to try and lose weight, but produce a lean body and a happy mind. The same principles of creating comfort when in pain apply to weight loss as well. Trying to lose weight is focusing on what you want to be rid of. Focus and image a lean, happy and healthy body, mind, and spirit. Use your Mind-Swords to give you new life.

Weight Loss Script

Now this script has the female pronoun. If you are male then simply change it for yourself.

Induction
Deepener

"...and now continue relaxing...drifting and dreaming... knowing that you are getting out of this pleasant state of relaxation exactly what you came here for.

For you want to be lean and healthy, you want to feel happier, more settled, more confident and most importantly you want to (insert your goals/motivations). And as a result of allowing yourself to relax so very well you are finding that all of these things are happening to you now.

So now, I want you to form a mental picture in your mind... I want you to picture as clearly as you can a five-storied Asian temple. If you cannot see the temple clearly, do not concern yourself, just continue relaxing and allow time to pass.

At the bottom gate of the temple you can see a woman who is very overweight, at least 20 pounds more than you. She too is a martial artist, but one who desires to be leaner and healthier than she is now.

See that woman at the bottom gate looking very sad and unhappy, and she is sad and unhappy as a result of her weight. She is aware that she lacks confidence in herself as a result of her weight. She feels unhealthy and gets out of breath so very easily. She feels unattractive, unwanted and (insert negative feelings taken from your list of reasons why you want to lose weight)

She is a sad and unhappy and feels that nothing in life is as happy as it should be because she is so overweight and out of shape.

See her looking up at the top of the temple and become aware, just as she does, that the temple is symbolic of her sadness and her overweight. The temple represents the difficulty she has in losing weight. She can also see on each floor of the temple, a guardian of that floor. These guardians are barriers that she has to face and must overcome to reach the fifth floor, the top of the temple.

So now, see her continuing to look at the top of the temple and as she does so, she can see another woman standing at the top of the temple, on the fifth floor.

The woman she sees has a trim, attractive, athletic figure. She is smiling and she is wearing her martial uniform that shows off her new figure and she feels proud. She is lean, healthy, full of life and enjoys life to the fullest. She is envied by other women because of her trim, muscular figure and because she too was once overweight, but through determination and effort, entered the temple, fought the guardians contained on each floor, climbed to the top of the temple, losing weight as she did so.

Her partner admires her and has nothing but praise for her. She... (Here include your picture of benefits for losing weight). She is a happy, confident woman.

Now look again at the woman at the bottom gate of the temple, see how sad, unhappy and miserable she is. See how she lacks confidence in herself.

Now once again look at the woman at the top tier of the temple, see how happy and confident she is.

Now once again see the woman at the bottom of the temple and as you do so you can see her gaining determination, strength, and confidence. She is beginning to feel strong and determined, determined to become lean and healthy, to fight her way to the top of the temple. See her entering the temple now.

And as she enters the temple see her facing the guardian of the first floor, see her easily dispatch the guardian and continues up to the second tier. See her defeat each floors' guardian, and she is finding it easier the higher she climbs, because as she dispatches each floors' guardian, she is getting leaner...and as she climbs she is getting stronger, fitter, leaner, healthier, and more confident. The higher she climbs, the leaner she gets, the stronger she gets and the more confidence she gains.

Now see her reach the top floor of the temple. See her standing next to the happy woman at the top of the temple. Notice how similar they look—both slim, lean, healthy and athletic. Now become aware that both women are beginning to look so much alike that they are as identical twins. And now I want you to merge the two women together into one. They are now one person, looking happy and confident.

Now become aware that the woman at the top tier of the temple is now you and that is where you want to be and deserve to be.

Now feel the strength and confidence of that woman. Feel the happiness, the sense of achievement. Keep these feelings with you and feel the determination to become lean and healthy growing stronger within you. Know deep down within yourself that you can defeat the guardians at each floor and reach the top, and that you want to reach the top of the temple and that you will do battle and reach the top of the temple.

And because you have allowed yourself to drift and dream and relax so very well, you are finding that the subconscious part of your mind that has been responsible for keeping you at the bottom of the temple will now do everything that it can to help you reach the top of the temple. Right to the very top. The subconscious mind knows that you will feel happier when you are lean, healthy, trim, and athletic. And because your subconscious mind wants you to be happy, you are finding that as from now, every day you are becoming leaner, and to help you to become lean and healthy this is what is happening to you.

Firstly, you are finding that at each and every meal a smaller amount of food is sufficient for you. Yes, a smaller amount of food is sufficient for you and as a result you are finding that at the end of each and every meal, no matter how little you have eaten, you are feeling comfortable full. At the end of each and every meal you are feeling comfortably full.

Yes, you are finding that at each and every meal a smaller amount of food is sufficient for you. Yes, a smaller amount of food is sufficient for you and as a result you are finding that at the end of each and every meal, no matter how little you have eaten, you are feeling comfortably full. At the end of each and every meal you are feeling comfortably full.

Yes, you are finding that at each and every meal a smaller amount of food is sufficient for you. Yes, a smaller amount of food is sufficient for you and as a result you are finding that at the end of each and every meal, no matter how little you have eaten, you are feeling comfortably full. At the end of each and every meal you are feeling comfortably full.

You are also finding that before you eat any foods you know are fattening or unhealthy foods, foods that prevent you from being lean and healthy, you are saying to yourself, "Hi there craving for unhealthy food, come watch me eat or drink something lean and healthy."

Yes, your are finding that before you eat any foods you know are fattening or unhealthy foods, foods that prevent you from being lean and healthy, you are saying to yourself, "Hi there craving for unhealthy food, come watch me eat or drink something lean and healthy."

Yes, your are finding that before you eat any foods you know are fattening or unhealthy foods, foods that prevent you from being lean and healthy, you are saying to yourself, "Hi there craving for unhealthy food, come watch me eat or drink something lean and healthy."

And because your desire to lose weight, to fight your way to the temple top, is far, far stronger than the desire to eat fattening or unhealthy foods, you are finding that without really thinking about it, you are finding it easy to refuse to eat foods that will prevent you from reaching the temple top, and becoming lean and healthy.

You are also finding that your desire to exercise, to practice your martial art, increasing every day. You find it enjoyable, knowing this will help you to reach the top of the temple and become lean and healthy.

Yes, you are also finding that your desire to exercise, to practice your martial art, increasing every day. You find it enjoyable, knowing this will help you to reach the top of the temple and become lean and healthy.

Yes, you are also finding that your desire to exercise, to practice your martial art, increasing every day. You find it enjoyable, knowing this will help you to reach the top of the temple and become lean and healthy.

And all these things happening to you every day is helping you to not only become lean and healthy, but also to feel happier, more content, more accepted, stronger, mentally and physically stronger and more optimistic in every way.

Now in a few moments time.....

Terminate session

*Eisan asked the old monk,
"I am off to war. Any advice?"*

The old monk replied, "Pay attention."

CHAPTER 20
The Way Home

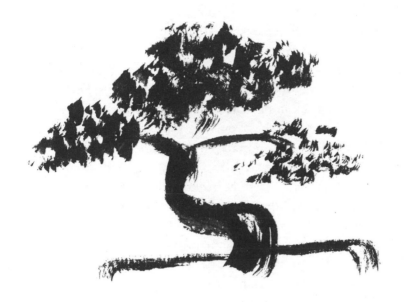

I have a friend, Scott, who runs a bookstore, called *The Way Home*.
It is a store filled with wonderful music, books, and conversation.
Whenever you go there, it feels like home. Scott makes you feel
comfortable as he walks up to you in his bright Hawaiian shirt and
Jerry Garcia looks. Without you feeling like he is a burden, Scott
asks how you are doing, and if you need any assistance. When you
tell him what your interests are, if there is someone in the store with
the same interests he connects you with that person, or he directs you
to the section of the store you will find most intriguing. It is a great
place to be. There is always hot tea, coffee, and the pleasant aroma of
temple incense, not to mention the calming sounds of gentle music
floating through the air.

By now it is my hope you have been able to find some relief from pain and suffering with the principles and practices found in *Black Belt Healing*. It is also my hope that you eventually come into contact with that state of mind, body, and spirit that gives you rest and the feeling you are finally home. As you know, there is no place like home. It is our refuge and place of peace. On a deep subconscious level there is a home that exists in all of us just waiting to be visited.

If you can recall, earlier in this book, I mentioned the road to becoming a black belt is paved with pain, and it is almost unimaginable to have earned one without it. But where does this road of pain take you after you have achieved your second, third, fourth degree black belts? I believe it is the road that is leading you home…and pain is the messenger beckoning you to return. Pain wakes you up to the reality of now and teaches you that the only way to move beyond pain is to travel on and embrace it. Yes, it does sound a bit crazy, but if you reflect upon this carefully, I believe you will eventually agree with me. Pain is the messenger beckoning you to that place of peace hidden deep within. All you have to do pay attention, listen, and take one step at a time.

To help guide you on your journey home, I have one more quick Mind-Sword technique for you to practice. As you are reading this, recall for a moment, perhaps after you have taken a long vacation or have been on an arduous journey, the time and place of finally arriving home. See yourself walk in the front door and put down your luggage. You go sit in your favorite easy chair, kick off your shoes, and settle into the soft cushions of your chair. Taking a great sigh of relief, feeling your chest rise and fall, you can now rest, you are home. Now anchor this feeling by touching a spot between your eyes, perhaps at the bridge of your nose or if you desire a little higher. Now whenever you need to feel at home, just touch that spot…and remember.

Thank you for taking the time in exploring the healing world of Mind-Swords Hypnosis.

May you find your way home.

Hands, palm to palm.

Appendix

A: Keeping it Legal

If you decide to help others manage their pain, and charge a fee, it is important that you, the hypnotist, adhere strictly to non-medical educational language and terminology. Refrain from any diagnostic or prescriptive references that could be misconstrued as "practicing medicine." The following information came from the Clayton College of Natural Health in the first chapter I ever read. This information is important for all of us who use Healing methods.

• You will want to use educational language which is always informative and empowering. It involves clearly increasing the client's knowledge regarding health, hypnosis and how the mind and body works. In that way, it empowers the client to make decisions and take greater responsibility about daily lifestyle and health choices for his or her own body, life, and health concerns.

• Diagnostic language includes any statement that sounds as though the hypnotherapist is telling the client what his/her problem or health issue might be.

- Prescriptive language is any information that the practitioner may offer that tells the client what to do (take Vitamin C) or how to do it, how often (three times per day), how much or what to do to "cure" the client.

Example: A client reports: "My knee hurts. It has been hurting every once in a while ever since I injured it doing some heavy bag work in the dojo. I am tired of pain killers. What else can I do?"

A diagnostic response would be: "You probably tore the medial meniscus." Or, "Arthritis could be setting in."

A prescriptive response would be: "Listen to this CD three times a day and this will decrease the swelling in our knee and the pain will subside."

An educational response would be: "Some of my other clients have reported that by listening to this pain management CD they have reduced their swelling in their joints and have decreased their pain."

If a client presents with a formal diagnosis from a medical professional still avoid prescriptive or diagnostic statements. It is imperative that you use educational language throughout your sessions as well as having all of your forms, notes, and materials in an educational format. This will keep you out of trouble on both legal and ethical arenas.

It is not illegal to inform and educate about good health and behavior change, yet the interpretation of how the information is conveyed can make the difference between being viewed by some as "practicing medicine without a license" or not. Educating and empowering the client is the ultimate goal of the hypnotherapist. Practice with a high level of professionalism and competency.

B: The Truth about Certification

If you wish to become certified in Mind-Swords Hypnosis, visit my web-site at www.blackbelthealing.com for information on my individualized mentorship/certification process.

The certification process is simple and based on a personalized mentorship model, similar to the "uchi deshi" model in martial arts. You will be trained in Hypnosis' three major areas of expertise...Pain Management, Weight Loss, and Smoking Cessation.

Whether you are a "white belt" in the use of hypnosis or already have an extensive background, feel free to contact me to set up your personalized program.

But before you choose to become certified I want you to be aware of certification and all that it holds. As a teacher of the martial arts I believe it is best to be open and honest about the nature of certification in hypnosis and hypnotherapy.

As you may or may not be aware of, presently there is NO form of federal regulation for hypnotherapy professionals. Plus, there are very few state and local regulations or laws governing the practice of hypnotherapy in the United States. It is important to check with your state and local government regarding the laws or regulation in operating a hypnotherapy practice.

It is also important to make sure that whoever "certifies" you is legitimate. There are many scam artists on the Internet who will certify you by just sending them a check. It is like getting a professional degree or martial rank via a diploma mill. This will come back and haunt you. Please be careful.

People that I certify will have the confidence knowing they have undergone professional training and are ready and able to be known as Black Belt Healers. Your clients will thank you as well.

C: Resources and Recommended Reading

If you are like me you love to read. Here are some of the books that have influenced my thought and perspectives of the world. I hope you enjoy them as well.

Aitken, Robert. *The Gateless Barrier.* San Francisco: North Point Press, 1990.

Brazier, David. *Zen Therapy.* New York: John Wiley and Sons, 1995.

Chodron, Pema. *The Wisdom of No Escape.* Boston: Shambhala Publications, 1991.

Chowaney, Nonin. *Nebraska Zen Center Sutra Book.* Omaha, NE: Nebraska Zen Center, 1992.

Funakoshi, Gichin. *Karate-do Nyumon: The Master Introductory Text.* Trans: by John Terausto. Tokyo: Kodansha International, 1988

Kabat-Zinn, Jon. *Full Catastrophe Living.* New York: Bantam Doubleday Dell Publishing, 1990

Katagiri, Dainin. *Returning to Silence.* Boston: Shambhala Publications, 1988.

LeCron, Leslie. *Self-Hypnotism: The Techniques and Its Use in Daily Living.* Englewood Cliffs, NJ: Pearson Ptr, 1964.

Reps, Paul. *Zen Flesh, Zen Bones.* Rutland, VT: Tuttle Publishing, 1985

Study Guide. "Keeping It Legal." Birmingham, AL: Clayton College of Natural Health, 2000.

Suzuki, Shunryu. *Zen Mind, Beginner's Mind.* New York: Weatherhill, Inc. 1970